A Colour Atlas of Clinical Orthopaedics

Copyright © L. Kessel, 1980
Published by Wolfe Medical Publications Ltd, 1980
Printed by Smeets-Weert, Holland
ISBN 0 7234 1546 3
Paperback edition, © 1988

A CIP catalogue record for this book is available from the British Library.

For a full list of Wolfe Medical Atlases, plus forthcoming titles and details of
our surgical, dental and veterinary Atlases, please write to Wolfe Medical
Publications Ltd, 2-16 Torrington Place, London WC1E 7LT, England.

A Colour Atlas of
Clinical Orthopaedics

Lipmann Kessel

MBE MC FRCS
Professor of Orthopaedics
Institute of Orthopaedics
Royal National Orthopaedic Hospital
London

Uta Boundy

Department of Medical Photography
Institute of Orthopaedics
London

Wolfe Medical Publications Ltd

Contents

Acknowledgements

I should like to thank my colleagues, past and present, on the staff of the Royal National Orthopaedic Hospital and the Institute of Orthopaedics (London) for their help in the use of much of the material in this Atlas. Thanks are also due to the following for permission to publish: Dr Barbara Ansell (figure **118**); Mr G. L. W. Bonney (figure **394**); Dr Mercer Rang (figure **133**); Dr Gerald Stern (figure **189 & 190**), and the Medical Photographic Departments, not only of the Institute of Orthopaedics, but also of St Bartholomew's, Charing Cross and University College Hospitals in London. Dr Paul Byers has given me considerable assistance in the legends to photomicrographs. Veronica Aurens has helped with the selection of radiographs; Ruth Campbell and Pat Sugden found obscure clinical records; and above all Betty Walton displayed great patience and expertise in the preparation of the manuscript. I extend my grateful thanks to all of them.

Uta Boundy, medical photographer at the Institute of Orthopaedics, who has collaborated throughout in the preparation of the manuscript, is acknowledged on the flyleaf.

1 Generalised disorders

One of the fascinations of clinical orthopaedic practice is to detect the patient who presents with an obvious local deformity or disability, which in the event turns out to be an expression of some generalised disease process. It is important that the clinician's attention is not overwhelmed by the local presenting disorder but that he remains aware of the fact that he may be seeing only the tip of an iceberg. Sometimes the generalised nature of the disease is obvious. At other times, e.g. a child presents with knock-knees who is in fact suffering from some form of rickets; or a child in whom the spinal curvature turns out to be the local manifestation of generalised neurofibromatosis.

The clinician should be on his guard lest the part which the patient presents to him, obscures the whole picture.

Achondroplasia

Developmental disorders of the skeleton may broadly be divided into those which give rise to dwarfism and those which do not. Classical achondroplasia is of autosomal dominant inheritance. The condition is either apparent at birth, or soon after. The abnormal skull and short limbs are characteristic. Physical strength and intelligence are *not* impaired.

1

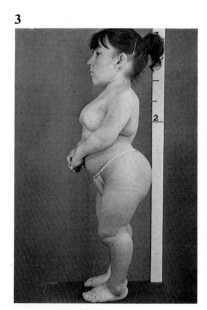

2

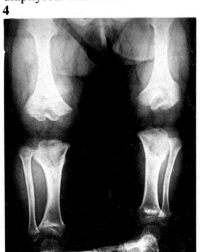

1–5 These strong little dwarfs are of typical appearance. Radiographs of the spine show flattening of the antero-superior aspect of the lumbar vertebra and widening of the intervertebral spaces in the lateral view. In the antero-posterior view there is progressive decrease in the interpedicular distances. Radiographs of the extremities show the characteristic 'ball in socket' epiphyses and flared metaphyses. The bones are short, giving an impression of diaphyseal thickness.

3

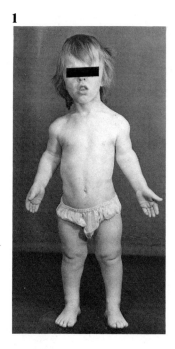

4

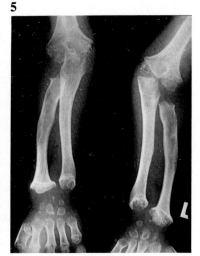

5

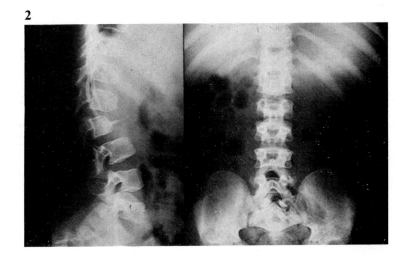

Enchondromatosis (dyschondroplasia – Ollier's disease)

No hereditary background is known, but dwarfism is common with disparity of growth between paired limbs. The affected limbs are short. These radiographs of a hand show multiple enchondromatosis.

6–10   This patient shows the typical disparity of growth of the arms.

6

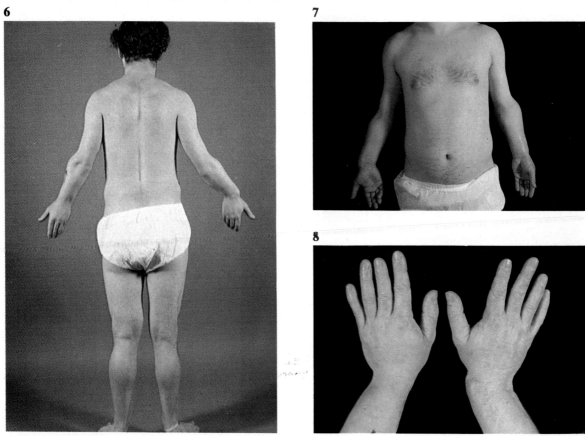

7

8

9 & 10   The radiographs show multiple enchondromata of the hands and disturbance of growth leading to deformity at the lower end of the radius.

9

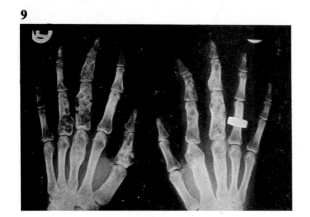

10

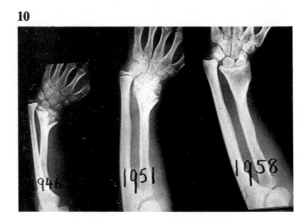

Diaphyseal aclasis (multiple hereditary exostoses)

A disorder of bone growth, giving rise to cartilage-capped exostoses which point away from the joint. This is of autosomal dominant inheritance and is very rarely associated with dwarfism.

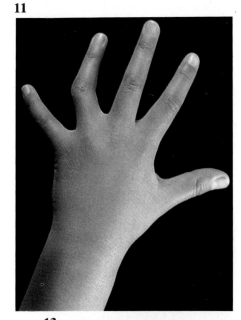

11–15 Although the disorder usually affects the lower limbs, any long bone may be involved. Angulation of the left ring finger has been caused by a cartilage-capped exostosis at the distal end of the proximal phalanx.

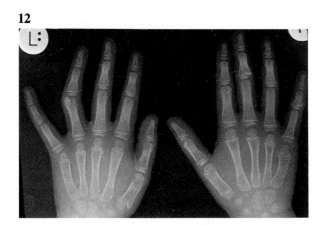

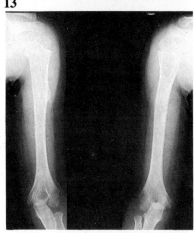

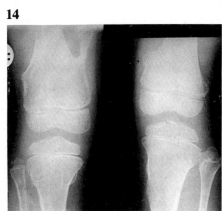

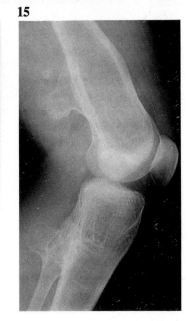

14 & 15 The exostosis always projects away from the adjacent joint. The exostosis is always capped by cartilage and therefore actually larger than seen on the radiograph.

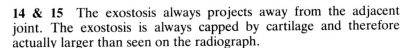

Spondylo-epiphyseal dysplasia

A comparatively rare type of generalised developmental disorder with a variety of autosomal patterns of inheritance. Characteristically, the trunk is short with scoliosis. Only the large proximal joints (hips and shoulders) are affected. Progressive scoliosis usually develops and premature degenerative arthritis of the hips and shoulders may occur, but the expectation of life is unaffected.

16

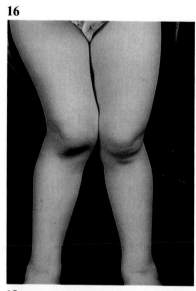

17

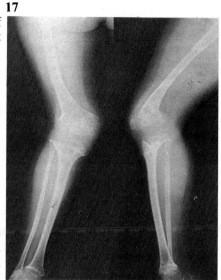

16–19 The disorder of growth-plate development causes deformity of the limb.

The vertebral end-plates are deformed and the vertebral bodies consequently distorted causing scoliosis to develop.

18

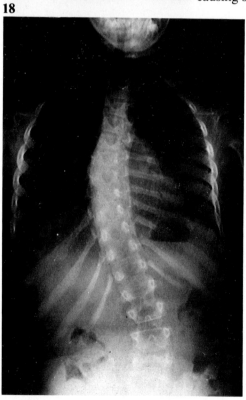

19

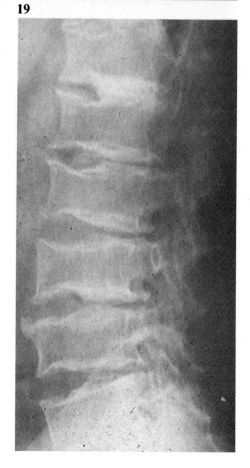

Metaphyseal dysostosis

A rare disorder of autosomal dominant inheritance. There is severe growth disturbance of the metaphyses of the long bones, obvious deformity and joint dysfunction. Two types have been described here:

20

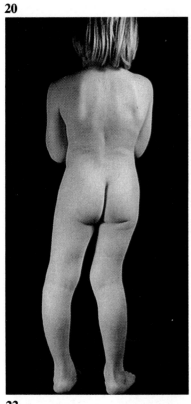

21

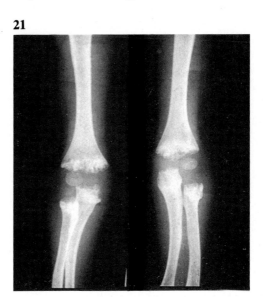

20 & 21   The Schmid type is relatively benign and occurs during infancy.

22

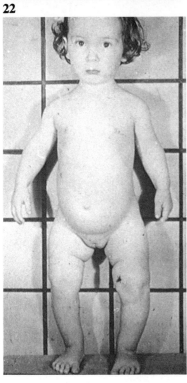

23

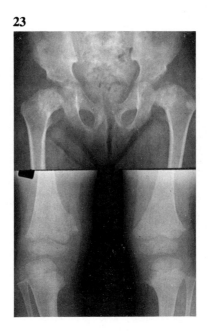

22 & 23   The Jansen type is apparent at birth and more severe.

Dysplasia epiphysealis hemimelica (Trevor's disease)

This is more common in the lower than in the upper limbs, usually on the medial side of the ankle or wrist.

24

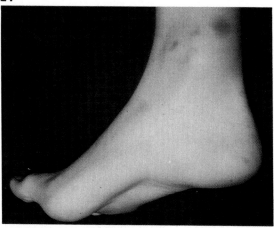

25

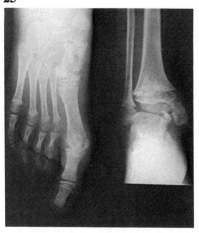

24 & 25 **A calcified mass** shown in radiographs of the ankle simulating a cartilage-capped exostosis, hypertrophied medial malleolus and medial cuneiform, and the whole of the first metatarsal ray. This disease presents with limitation of movement and some pain.

26

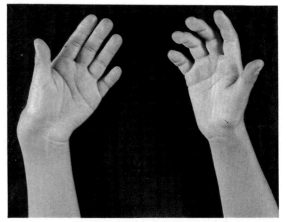

27

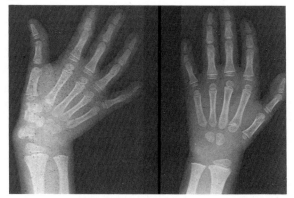

26 & 27 **Radial enlargement and ulnar deviation** of the left wrist of this ten-year-old boy is clinically obvious. The radiographs show considerable precocity of maturation of the carpus as well as the development of bosses of new bone simulating ossified chondromata.

Phocomelia

The thalidomide disaster has again drawn attention to the possible serious consequences of noxious intra-uterine influences on the foetus. Maternal infection by rubella as well as the use of Thalidomide during pregnancy are probably only the most obvious and serious examples.

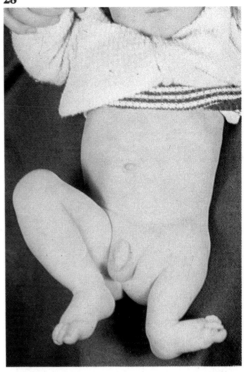

28–30 The boy shown in figures 29 and 30 is of normal intelligence and well developed in all respects except that his upper limbs have failed to develop. He has no left arm and his right arm consists of a little flipper (*G.phoke*, seal; *melos*, limb). The infant shown in figure 28 is normal apart from a failure in development of the left lower limb.

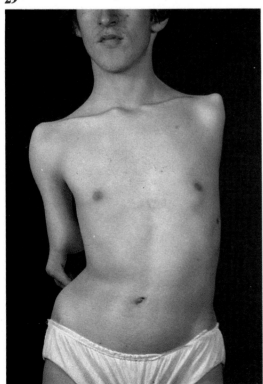

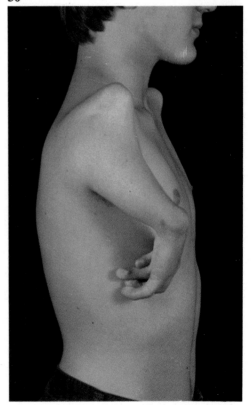

Osteogenesis imperfecta (brittle bones)

This condition usually occurs sporadically, but may be an autosomal dominant. There is generalised disturbance of connective tissue development, including bone. Blue sclera and imperfect dentition are noted. There are two types: *congenita* and *tarda*. Both are characterised by frequent fractures, often multiple, leading to distortion of growth in all planes. Renal calculi occur due to the rapid turnover of bone.

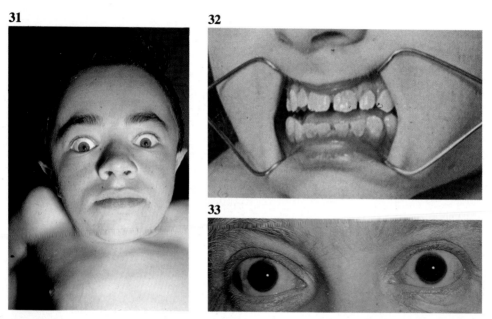

31–33 Blue sclera and imperfect dentition.

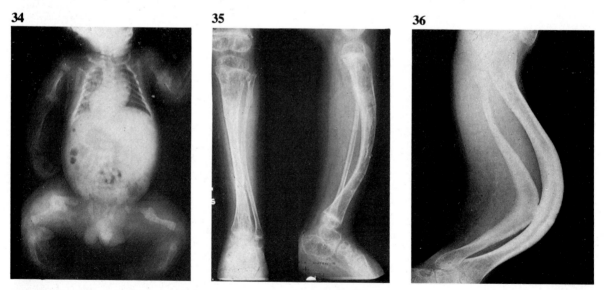

34–36 A general radiograph of the infant shows multiple fractures. If the child survives, the frequent fractures cause gross distortion of the long bones.

Arthrogryposis multiplex congenita

There is absence of muscle development around the joints, which are consequently stiff and contracted. The commonest type, which is depicted here, affects the lower limbs only. In about 10 per cent of cases the upper limbs alone are affected, whilst in 30 per cent of cases both upper and lower limbs are affected. The condition occurs sporadically and is possibly associated with prolonged intra-uterine immobilisation of the foetus from a number of different causes. The mental condition is, however, normal.

37

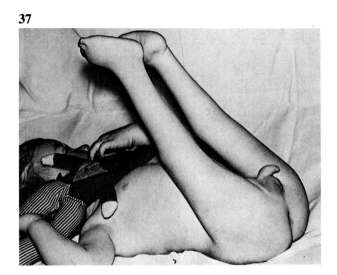

38

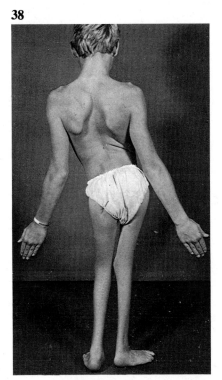

37–40 The commonest type of arthrogryposis multiplex congenita affecting the lower limbs only.

39

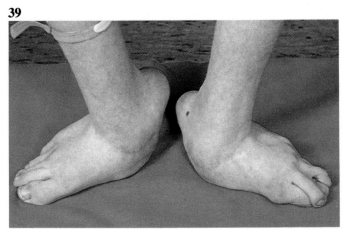

40

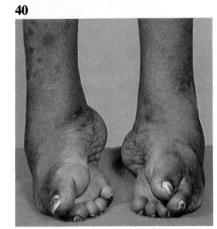

41

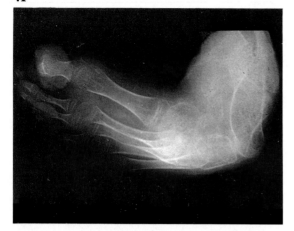

42

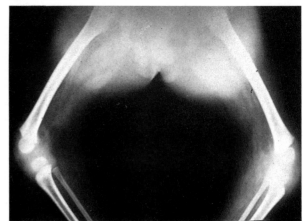

41 & 42 Arthrogryposis multiplex congenita. Radiographs show normal bone pattern but gross deformity of joints, which often includes dislocation. Radiographs of long bones show the diminished muscle mass and muscle pattern in the limbs.

43

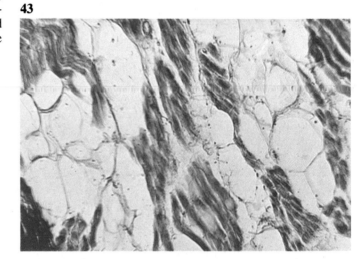

Histopathology shows fatty infiltration of muscle. *(× 75)*

Neurofibromatosis (von Recklinghausen's disease)

This is a syndrome of autosomal dominant inheritance which varies considerably in extent. There is characteristic pigmentation of the skin known as 'cafè-au-lait' patches. One or two isolated tumours of nerve trunks sometimes cause erosive changes of nearby bone. Widespread involvement of a single limb may give rise to hypertrophy and distortion of growth. The most serious skeletal manifestations of neurofibromatosis are scoliosis with serious distortion of vertebral growth and characteristic scalloping of the posterior aspects of vertebral bodies.

44 **45** **46**

47 **48** **49**

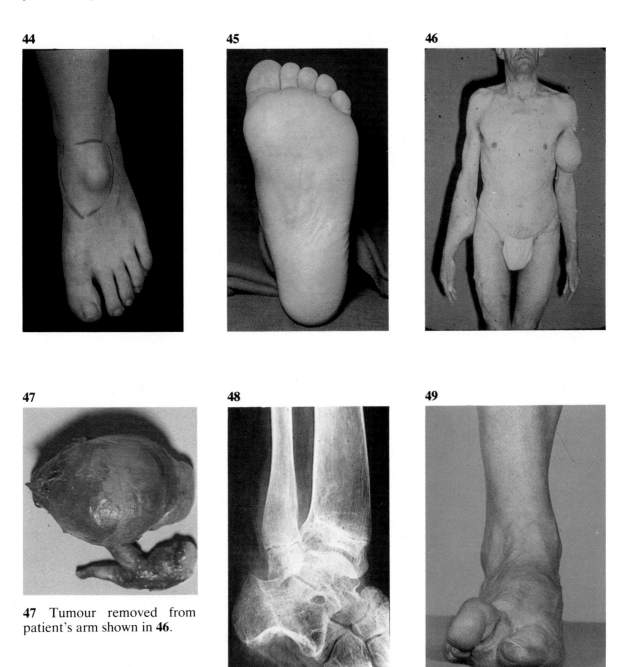

47 Tumour removed from patient's arm shown in **46**.

48 Erosion of the plantar aspect of the calcaneus due to an adjacent neurofibroma.

49 Hypertrophy of the second toe.

50 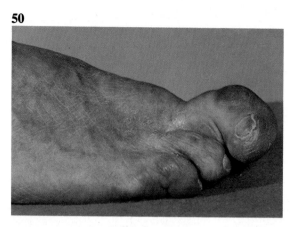   **51**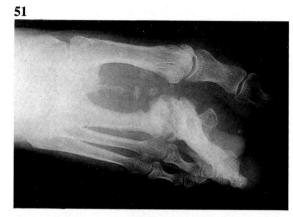

50 & 51   Gigantism of the third toe in a patient suffering from von Recklinghausen's disease.

52 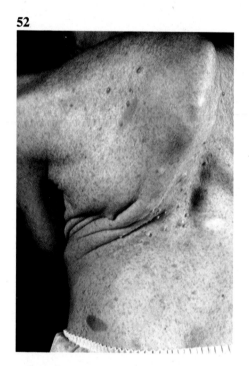   **53**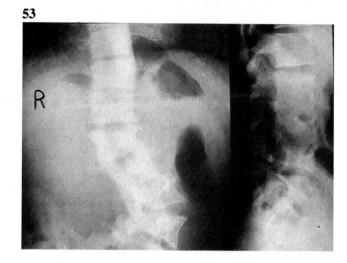

52 & 53   Pigmentation of the skin, and multiple neurofibromata of varying size, typical of von Recklinghausen's disease, which may be associated with severe scoliosis.

54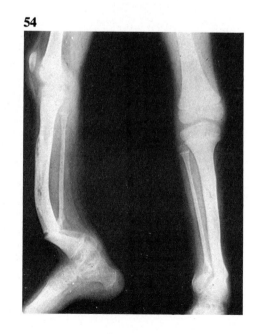

54   Pseudarthrosis of the tibia is another curious but serious skeletal association.

Ehlers-Danlos syndrome

Excessive mobility of the joints or being 'double-jointed' varies from comparatively mild ligamentous laxity, expressed in an ability to hyperextend the knee, elbow, wrist, and fingers, to a more severe disorder.

55

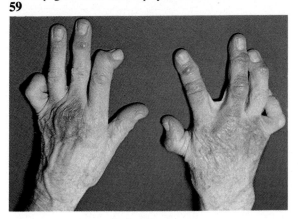

55   Excessive mobility of the joints.

56

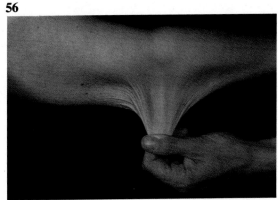

56   In the Ehlers-Danlos syndrome the excessive ligamentous laxity is only one aspect of a widespread connective tissue disorder expressed, for example, in hyperelasticity of the skin.

57

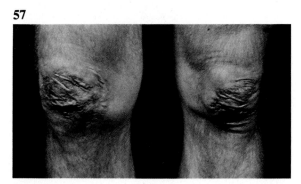

57   The skin has a tendency to split easily and leave pigmented tissue-paper scars.

58

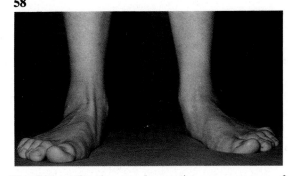

58   Ehlers-Danlos syndrome is a rare cause of flat-foot.

59

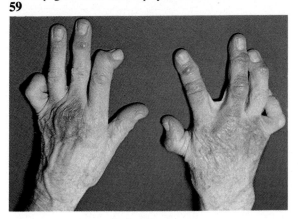

60

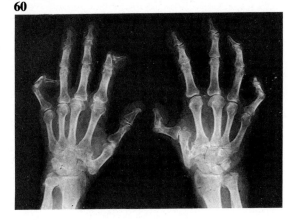

59 & 60   Destructive arthropathy, in which the carpometacarpal joint of the thumb is particularly affected, may eventually develop. Although the disease is rare, its importance lies in the associated cardiovascular disorders which are occasionally serious.

Haemophilia

61

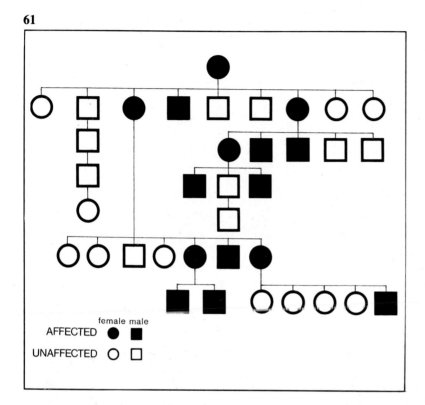

62

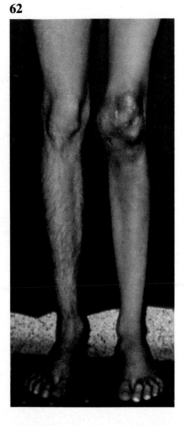

61 Queen Victoria's family tree.
Classical haemophilia is transmitted by the female and becomes manifest in the male. It is therefore of X-linked recessive inheritance. Apart from its obvious manifestations of excessive bleeding due to impairment of clotting factors in the blood, it may give rise to haemorrhagic tumours in muscle. Joints are damaged by repeated haemorrhage from trivial injuries.

62 Discolouration and swelling of the left knee due to repeated minor haemorrhagic incidents.

63

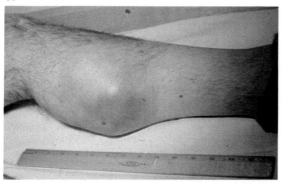

64

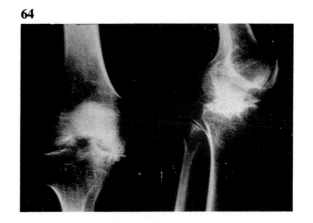

63   Haemorrhagic 'tumour' in the calf muscle.

65

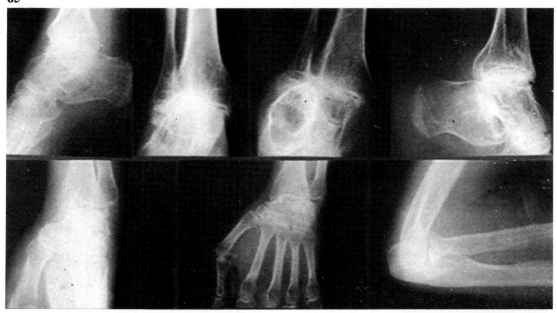

64–65   One or several joints become damaged by
repeated haemorrhage, and ultimately a destructive
form of arthropathy becomes manifest.

66

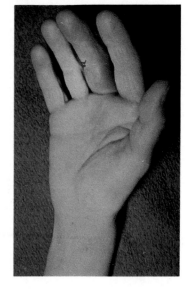

66   **Von Willebrand's disease.** Although by defini-
tion classical haemophilia cannot occur in women,
there is a rare dyscrasia of the blood-clotting
mechanism which does affect women, known as
von Willebrand's disease. The disease is much less
severe, and unlike haemophilia, petechiae of the
skin do occur in this disease.

Generalised osteoarthritis

Osteoarthritis is a degenerative process beginning in the articular cartilage and eventually involving the whole joint. Osteoarthritis should be regarded as secondary to a cause which careful search should disclose.

  All the cases of 'primary' generalised osteoarthritis as depicted here are probably secondary, although at present their cause or causes are unknown.

67–70 Primary generalised osteoarthritis is typified by the involvement of the terminal interphalangeal joints of the fingers in which Heberden's nodes can be seen on the dorsum of the joints.

67

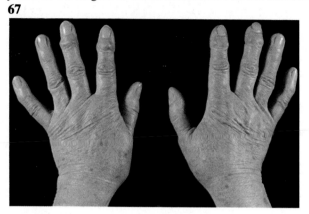

68

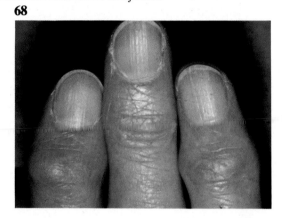

69 The terminal phalangeal joints are primarily affected.

69

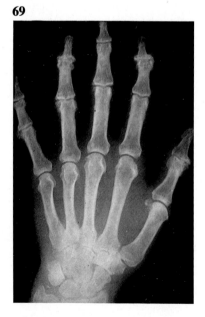

70 The carpometacarpal joint of the thumb is commonly afflicted.

70

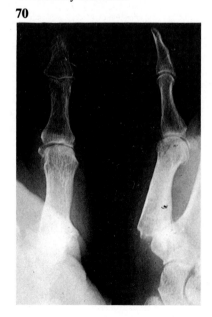

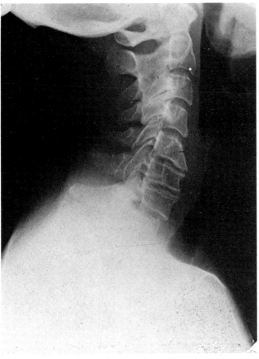

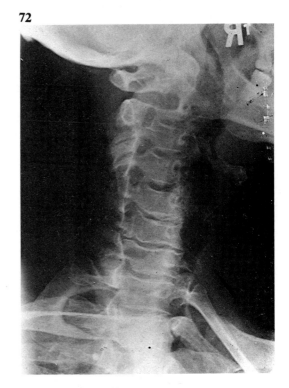

71 & 72 Cervical spondylosis: the complex of joints of the cervical spine are commonly affected.

There are a variety of causes of painful neck including a prolapsed cervical intervertebral disc, tuberculous or pyogenic infection, or tumours involving the vertebral column. By far the commonest, however, is osteoarthritis of the cervical spine (cervical spondylosis).

Although primary degenerative arthritis of the cervical spine can be initiated by injury, it is often simply a manifestation of generalised degenerative changes which occur with increasing age (see diagram **381**).

Degenerative osteoarthritis usually commences at the most mobile section of the neck, starting at C5/6 and moving downwards to involve the lowest three cervical joints. The changes affect first the intervertebral joints with accompanying disc degeneration, and later the postero-lateral facet joints. Osteophytes developing at the margin of the facet joints encroach upon the intervertebral foramina and irritate the emerging cervical nerve roots by direct pressure.

73   **74**   **75**

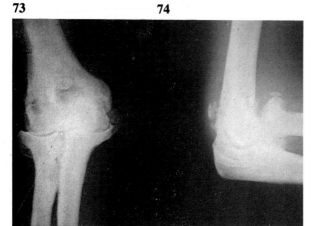

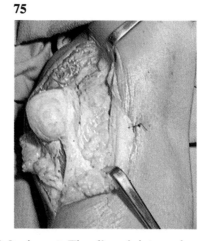

73-75   **Baker's cyst.** The elbow joints are less commonly affected by osteoarthritis. A synovial protrusion may develop, particularly in the elbow and the knee: a so-called Baker's cyst.

76   **77**

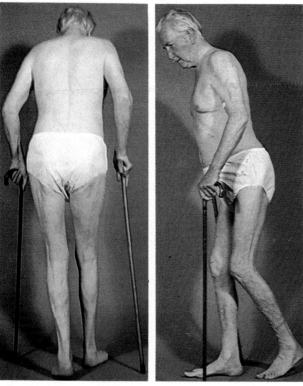

78

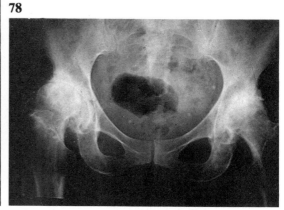

76–78   **Degenerative osteoarthritis.** This elderly gentleman requires two walking sticks to overcome the disability of painful, stiff and flexed hip joints. His radiograph shows the typical appearances of degenerative osteoarthritis – so-called primary osteoarthritis. Because the disease is so far advanced, any disorder of the hips which may have given rise to the arthritis is obscured by the severe changes which have developed later. There is loss of joint space due to loss of articular cartilage, sub-articular sclerosis of the bone on either side of the joint, and marginal osteophyte formation have occurred.

79

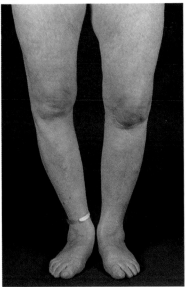

80

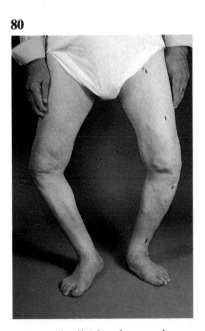

79–81 Osteoarthritis of the knees is only slightly less common. Genu varum gradually develops and may become very severe.

81

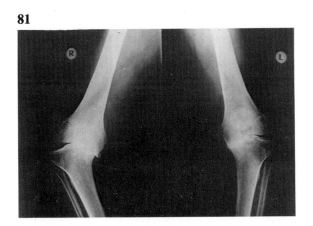

82

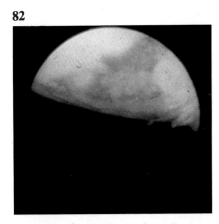

82 Arthroscopic view illustrates how the disease starts in the articular cartilage.

83

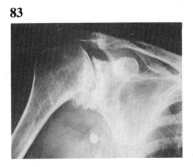

84

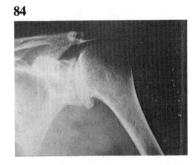

83 & 84 Severe degenerative osteoarthritis: in the shoulders of a 70-year-old lady, affecting both glenohumeral and acromio-clavicular joints. The cause of this osteoarthritis certainly can be guessed: it is calculated that she rowed some 1½ million strokes during 50 years rowing as a member of a ladies' rowing club!

Rheumatoid arthritis and related diseases

Rheumatoid arthritis is only the most obvious effect of general systemic rheumatoid disease and is probably caused by a number of factors, at present obscure. Our state of knowledge suggests that it may be due to an auto-immune response in a genetically susceptible individual. One of its more obvious orthopaedic manifestations is the enlargement of synovial-lined tissues such as bursae, tendon sheaths, and the synovial membrane of joints.

85

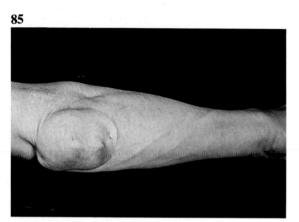

85   Olecranon bursitis.

86

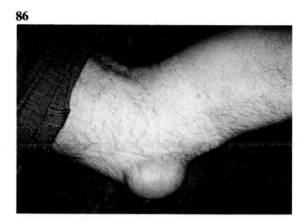

86   Prepatellar bursitis.

87

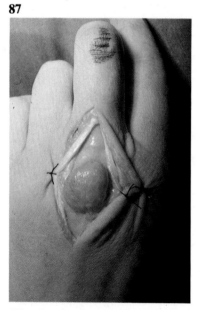

87   A single extensor tendon sheath of a finger is involved.

88

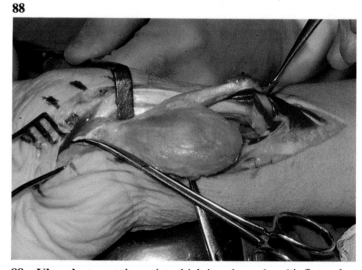

88   Ulnar bursa at the wrist which is enlarged and inflamed.

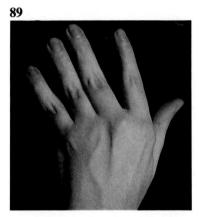

89 **Ulnar deviation** is often an early and characteristic deformity of the hand in rheumatoid arthritis.

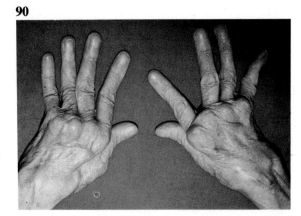

90 & 91 **Disorganisation of all the joints of the hands.** This affects principally the metacarpophalangeal joints and the proximal interphalangeal joints of the fingers in an advanced case.

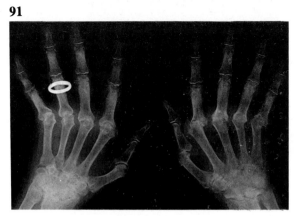

92 **'Swan-neck' deformity** of fingers due to rupture of the volar plate of PIP joints, or impediment of function of flexor sublimis.

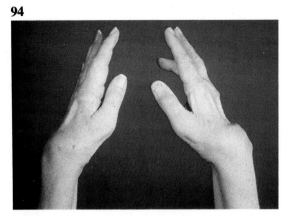

93 **Erosive arthropathy** of affected joints.

94 **Diseased synovial membrane** of the wrist showing hypertrophy.

95

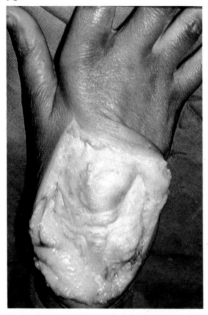

95 Inflamed synovial membrane of the extensor tendon sheaths at the wrist with hypertrophy.

96

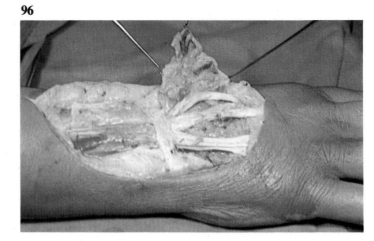

96 Surgical removal of the diseased synovial tissue.

97

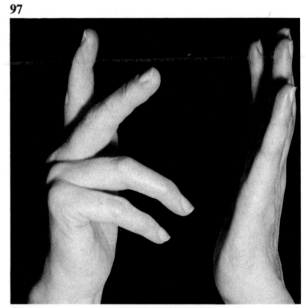

97 Rupture of extensor tendons due to synovial disease at the wrist causing 'dropped fingers'.

98

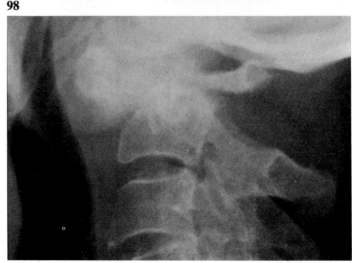

98 Subluxation of the atlas on the axis. Many patients with rheumatoid disease have lax ligaments of the joints of the cervical spine, leading to subluxation.

99

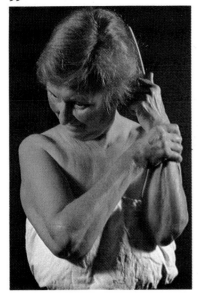

100

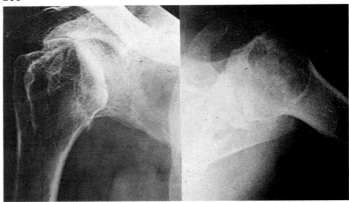

99 & 100   Rheumatoid arthritis of the shoulder joints. Rheumatoid disease is the only common cause of glenohumeral arthritis.

101

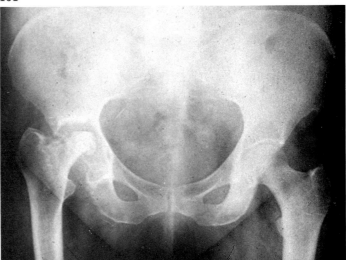

101 & 102   Destructive arthropathy of the hip joint produced by rheumatoid arthritis. This leads to erosions of the femoral head **102** and acetabulum.

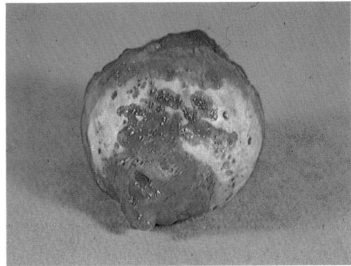

103

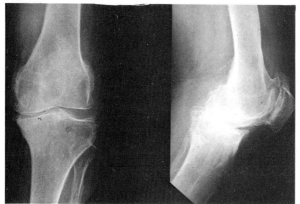

103 The knee joints are often affected.

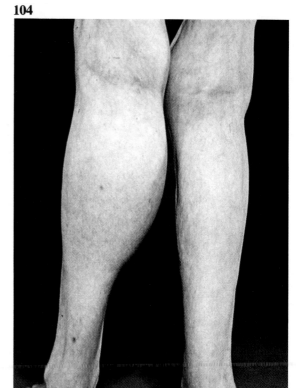

104 **Baker's cyst.** Enlargement of the calf in the same patient, due to diseased synovial membrane burrowing deeply from the joint into the calf, giving rise to a 'Baker's cyst'.

105 **Multiple synovial villi** in the knee of the same patient, seen through an arthroscope.

105

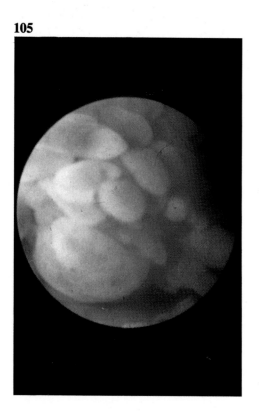

106

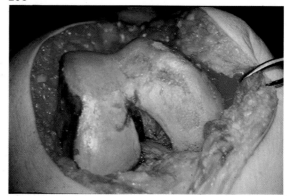

106 Loss of articular cartilage and general destructive arthropathy seen in the same patient at operation.

107

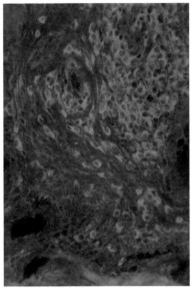

107 Rheumatoid synovial membrane prepared to show the immuno-fluorescence in the plasma cells.

108

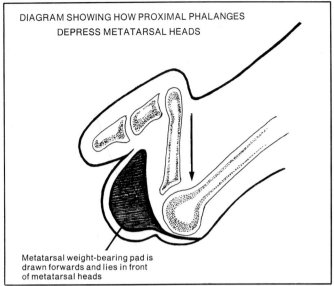

DIAGRAM SHOWING HOW PROXIMAL PHALANGES DEPRESS METATARSAL HEADS

Metatarsal weight-bearing pad is drawn forwards and lies in front of metatarsal heads

108 The metatarsal fat-pad is displaced forwards and the metatarsal heads become subcutaneous.

109

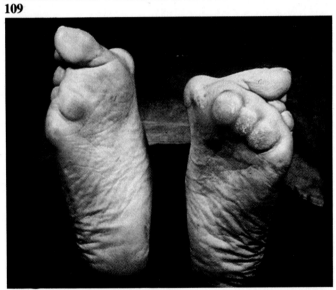

110

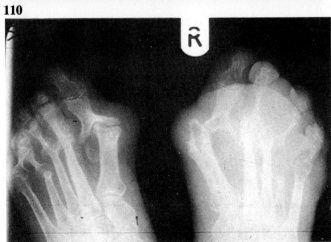

109 & 110 Rheumatoid arthritis may cause gross destructive arthropathy and distortion of the foot leading to painful callosities. Multiple subluxation and discoloration of the joints of the forefoot.

Ankylosing spondylitis

This condition is characterised by increasing pain and stiffness in the lumbar spine and buttocks, occasional vague pains elsewhere, e.g. in the heels, associated with general malaise and fatigue. The aetiology is unknown, but recent work suggests that there may be a genetic factor. The histocompatability antigen HLA-B27 is present in over 90 per cent of patients but in less than 10 per cent of the general population.

111

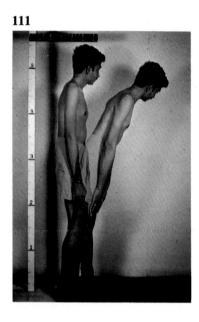

112

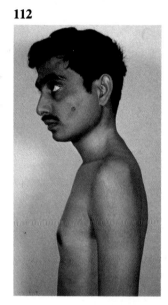

111 Gross loss of forward flexion on attempted toe-touching.

112 On attempting to turn his head the patient turns his eyes outwards, but his neck is held rigidly.

113

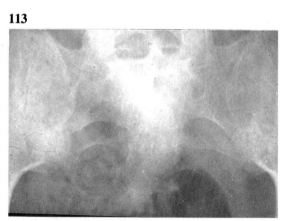

114

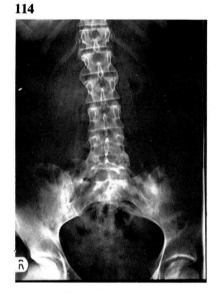

113 & 114 Apart from limited chest expansion and a raised ESR the earliest objective evidence is blurring and later, obliteration of the sacro-iliac joints.

115

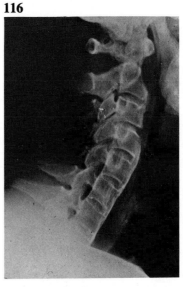

116

117

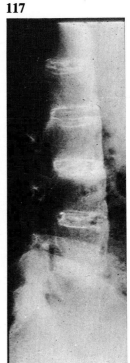

115 Eventually the trunk may become fixed in a fully bent position, so that the patient cannot see ahead.

116 & 117 'Bamboo spine'. Rigid bony and ankylosis of all major spinal joints.

Reiter's syndrome

The classical triad is of non-specific urethritis, conjunctivitis and arthritis.

118

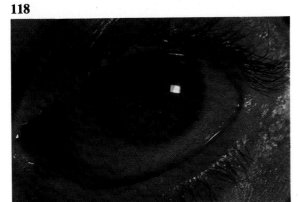

118 Subacute conjunctivitis in a case of Reiter's syndrome.

119

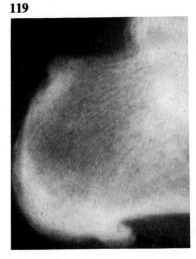

119 New bone formation producing spurs on the calcaneus.

120

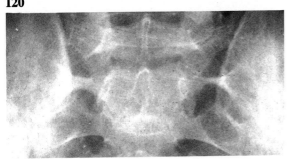

120 Blurring of joint space, marginal erosion and sclerosis of sacro-iliac joints typical of Reiter's syndrome.

Psoriatic arthropathy

There is a peculiar association between psoriasis and arthropathy which affects principally the joints of hands and feet, and rarely the large and more proximal joints, resembling rheumatoid arthritis.

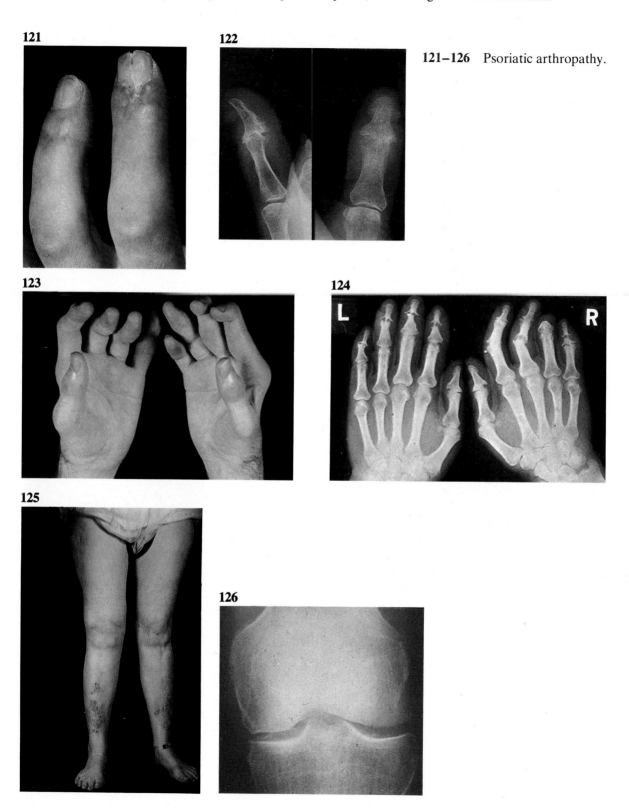

121

122

121–126   Psoriatic arthropathy.

123

124

125

126

Juvenile rheumatoid disease (Still's disease)

The illness corresponding to rheumatoid disease in adults. The joint changes are similar to those in adults but there is usually more severe general systemic illness.

127

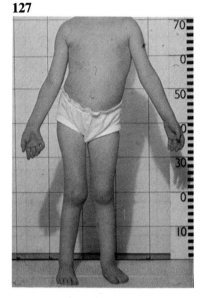

128

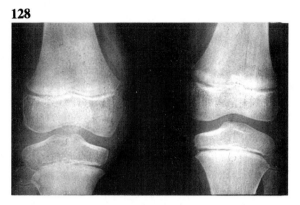

127 & 128   Early Still's disease in a child showing some swelling of the knee joints. The radiographs of the early stages show only soft tissue swelling with osteoporosis.

129

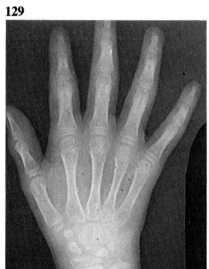

130

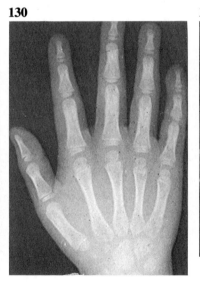

131

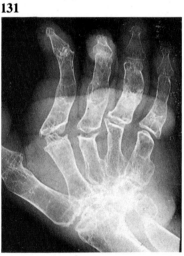

129 & 130   There is an enlargement of the growing ossific centres. Compare the radiographs of two children of the same age: on the left a child with Still's disease, on the right normal.

131   Enlargement of the shafts of the phalanges due to repeated periosteal reaction may occur.

132   The end result of a severe case. Deformity and spontaneous ankylosis has occurred. Such a serious result is the exception rather than the rule.

132

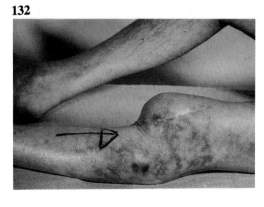

Infection of bone and joint

Acute pyogenic osteomyelitis and acute pyogenic arthritis, (which is almost always secondary to intra-articular osteomyelitis), was at one time very common, and even severe enough to be fatal.

The advent of antibiotics has completely altered the incidence of the disease, the course of the disease, and its destructive potential. The beneficial effects of early antibiotic therapy prevents many of the ghastly consequences of the infection, but does carry with it the problem of masking the early diagnosis.

Pyogenic osteomyelitis is almost always secondary to some distal focus such as a boil on the skin causing pyaemia. The commonest infecting organism is the *staphylococcus aureus,* but modern bacteriological techniques have displayed a wide range of potential infecting organisms, such as typhoid, salmonella, h.influenzae, etc. Even virus osteomyelitis, in particular the smallpox virus, has been found to cause acute and subsequently chronic infection of bone and joint. In tropical regions the range of infecting agents is correspondingly more extensive. Osteomyelitis caused by salmonella infection may occur in multiple foci, particularly in children or in patients suffering from sickle cell anaemia. Brucellosis is endemic in certain parts of the American mid-west, derived from pigs and cattle. For some unaccountable reason the vertebral column is involved in the vast majority of these patients.

Although the pathological reaction to infection in bone does not differ in essence from that in other tissues, it is considerably modified by the loss of blood supply to a bone due to endosteal infection when simultaneously an abscess has stripped off the periosteum. Even when the focus of infection has been sterilised by antibiotic therapy, the mineralised structure of bone creates special problems of healing which may lead to late development of sequestra in which an adequate concentration of antibiotics at the site of infection cannot be obtained. For this reason the early diagnosis, isolation of the infecting organism to test its precise sensitivity to antibiotics, and the relief of the tension of the abscess causing avascular bone necrosis, is imperative.

If treatment has been delayed or the initial treatment has not controlled the infection, a chronic bone abscess, a so-called Brodie's abscess, may develop. The abscess contains necrotic debris and bacterial colonies which are walled off by fibrous tissue and surrounding dense woven bone. Such an abscess may persist for years before it gives rise to symptoms.

Tuberculous osteomyelitis and arthritis run much the same course as the pyogenic disease but is usually less virulent at onset and more insidious in its clinical course. It is always secondary to some established focus of tuberculosis elsewhere in the body, commonly in the lungs or ileocaecal lymph nodes.

133 **Aspiration of pus** containing *staphylococcus pyogenes* from the hip-joint of an infant.

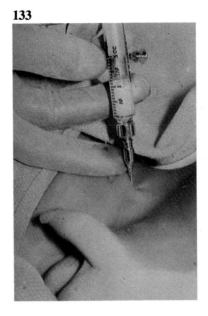

134 **135** **136**

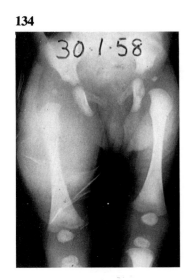 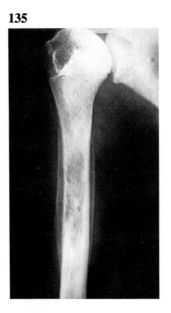 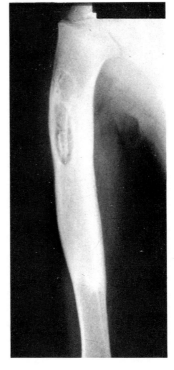

134–136 **Acute osteomyelitis** of a long bone from the stage of abscess formation in the metaphysis, (radiographically seen in the soft tissues only), ultimately leading to a localised obscess cavity containing a sequestrum of dead bone (Brodie's abscess).

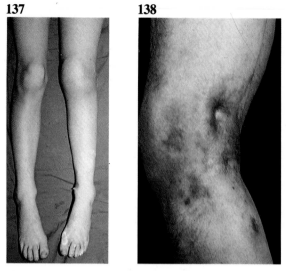

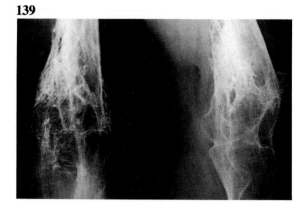

138 & 139 Bony ankylosis. The end result of a severe case of septic arthritis of the knee.

137 Septic arthritis of the knee-joint in an adolescent due to *staphylococcus pyogenes*.

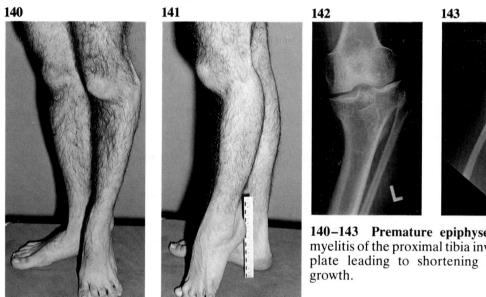

140–143 Premature epiphyseal arrest. Osteomyelitis of the proximal tibia involving the growth-plate leading to shortening and distortion of growth.

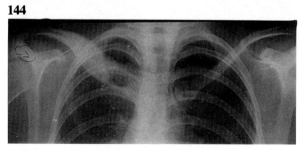

144 Chronic osteomyelitis of the clavicle. Repeated tests showed it to be due to *staphylococcus albus.*

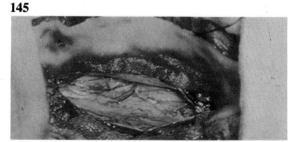

145 Intradural abscess containing *staphylococcus pyogenes* from a distant site. The patient was admitted with total paraplegia, but made a good recovery.

Tuberculous infection

Tuberculosis of bone or joint is the local manifestation of general disease, although it may be the most obvious and important presenting feature. The initial lesion is usually in lung or intestine, caused by the human or bovine tubercle bacillus. Formally 85 per cent were bovine in origin, but in the economically developed world where the disease is now very much less common, pasteurisation and TT testing (tuberculin) has reduced bovine cases to 25 per cent of the total. Orthopaedic hospitals in the 19th century were built in the countryside with the main object of treating tuberculosis of bone and joint in young people. The disease is now far less common, but is still occasionally seen either as an acute episode, or as the result of past infection. In the economically developing countries orthopaedic tuberculosis still presents a very serious problem. A few examples are shown here.

146

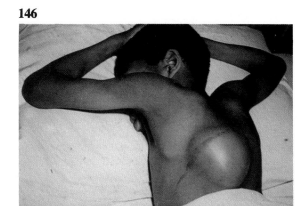

146   A 'cold' abscess in a child presenting in the loin as a painless swelling arises from infection of the spine.

147

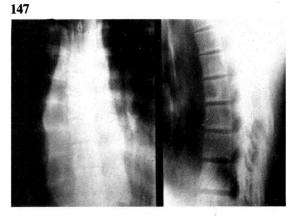

147   The tuberculous focus seen in the dorsal spine with its surrounding abscess formation.

148

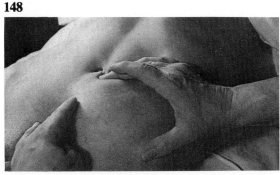

149

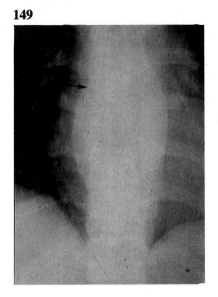

150

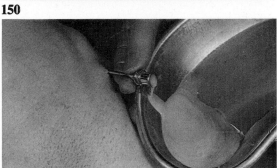

148–150   A cold abscess arising in the retro-peritoneal tissues from the dorsal spine may present as an abdominal mass.

151

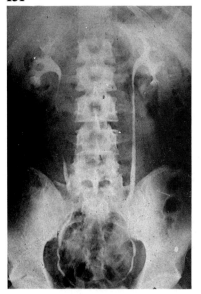

152

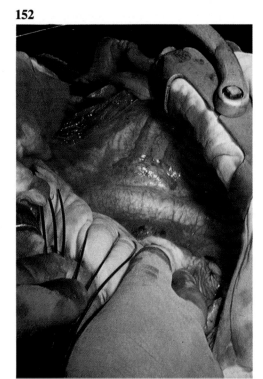

151 **The cold abscess** may lie within the sheath of the psoas muscle and may then present as a psoas abscess. An intravenous pyelogram shows the right ureter slightly obstructed and displaced by the psoas abscess.

152 **A tuberculous cold abscess of the dorsal spine** seen above the thoracic aorta at operation.

153

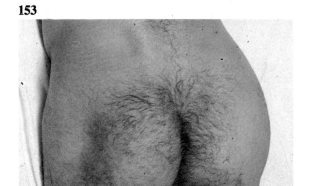

154

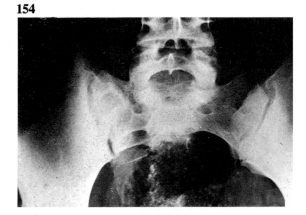

153 & 154 **Tuberculosis of the right sacro-iliac joint** presenting as a cold abscess in the buttock.

155

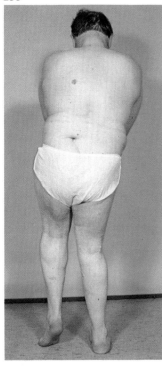

156

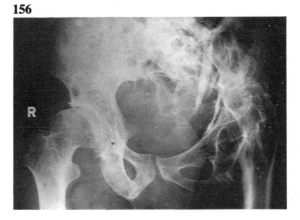

155 & 156 Old tuberculosis of the left hip joint
causing destruction and a fibrous ankylosis with
adduction deformity and shortening.

157

158

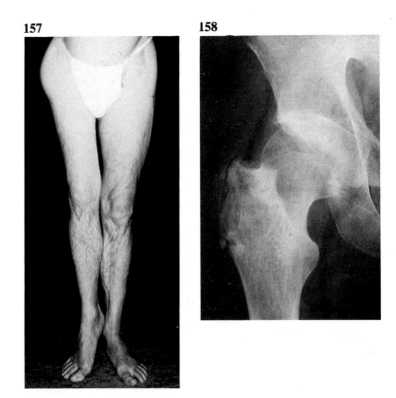

157 & 158   Tuberculosis of the trochanteric bursa.
The cold abscess is visible and palpable over the
greater trochanter, which is seen to be eroded.

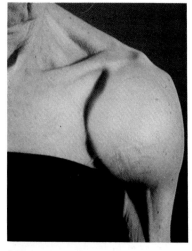

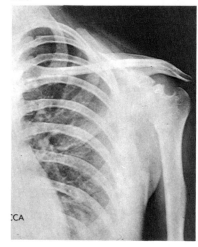

159 & 160 Tuberculosis of the shoulder joint with cold abscess formation. Sometimes tuberculosis occurs in the shoulder with little or no pus formation, and is called 'caries sicca'.

161

162

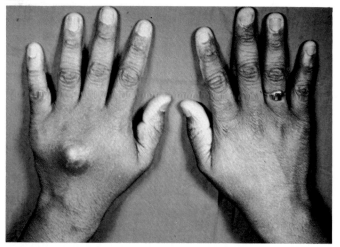

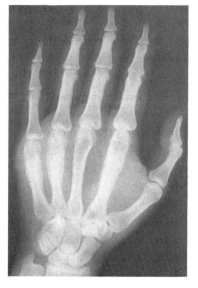

161 & 162 Tuberculous dactylitis. The focus is seen in the shaft of the fourth metacarpal bone of the left hand.

163

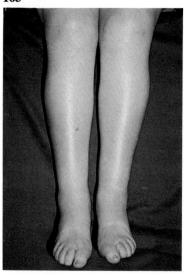

163 Scrofulous oedema. A case of longstanding tuberculous infection of the spine in which the lymphatic flow from the lower limbs is obstructed.

Neurology in orthopaedics

There is an intimate clinical relation between orthopaedics and neurology. Since neurology pervades almost the whole of orthopaedic surgery, only a few examples of the more immediate and obvious relation can be shown here.

The effects following poliomyelitis (APM) are extremely variable. Deformities are occasionally due to gravity, but principally depend on the imbalance of muscles. The stronger surviving muscles produce the deformity: a limb which is totally paralysed usually has no fixed deformity. Occasional limb-length inequality develops, particularly if the disease occurred in early childhood.

164 **Flail arm** following poliomyelitis in infancy.

165 **Paralytic subluxation of the shoulder.** There is obvious wasting of the deltoid.

164

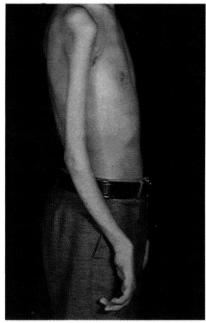

165

166

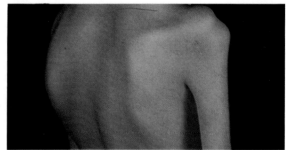

167

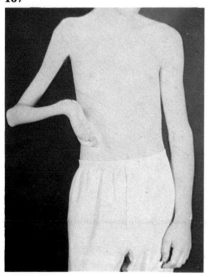

166 **Severe claw-hand.** Paralysis of the intrinsic muscles of the hand following poliomyelitis. The deformity is due to the fact that the long flexors and extensors of the fingers have *not* been affected. The claw-hand develops due to paralysis of their antagonists – the short intrinsic muscles.

167 **Poliomyelitis in infancy** affected only the right upper limb in this young man. Weak active abduction of the shoulder and flexion of the elbow are all that remain in this withered and almost flail arm.

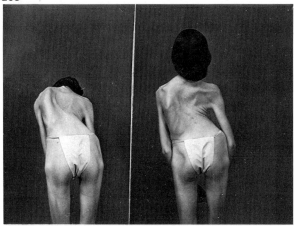

168 **Paralytic scoliosis** may follow poliomyelitis affecting the trunk muscles.

169 **Contracture of tensor fascia femoris muscle.** Because the muscle traverses both hip and knee it can produce flexion deformities at both joints.

169

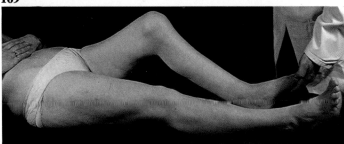

171

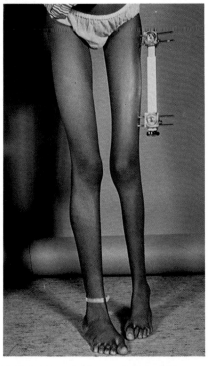

170

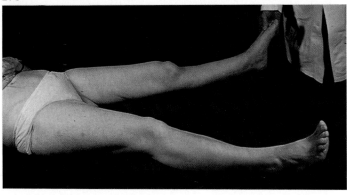

170 **Yount's test.** Both deformities of the hip and knee are corrected by simple abduction of the hip.

171 **Dropped foot (paralytic equinus).** Shortening of the left lower limb with equinus deformity of the ankle and foot. The equinus may be beneficial to compensate for the shortened leg. (The patient has a Wagner-type leg lengthening apparatus *in situ*.)

172

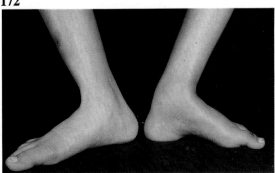

172 **Pes calcaneo-cavus:** the deformity is due to paralysis of the calf muscles.

173

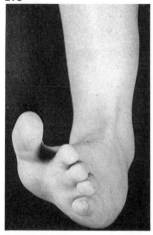

174

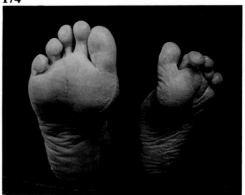

175

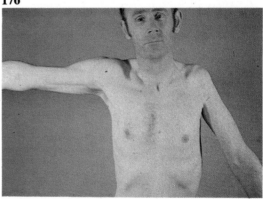

176

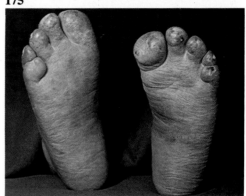

177

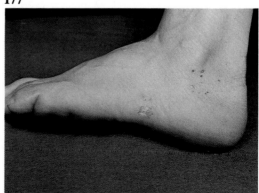

173 Weakness of tibialis anterior and the peroneal muscles. When he attempts to dorsiflex the ankle, the toes extend strongly in an attempt to compensate for the loss of ankle dorsiflexors. The deformity is due to the unbalanced action of normal extensor toe muscles acting in the presence of paralysed tibialis anterior and peroneal muscles.

174 The opposite deformity is demonstrated here: the peroneal muscles are the stronger surviving group. The foot therefore moves into forcible eversion with depression of the head of the first metatarsal by the unopposed action of a strongly contracting peroneus longus muscle.

175 Polio-paraplegia in a middle-aged woman, who suffered an attack of poliomyelitis in infancy. There is no active muscle in the lower limbs and therefore no significant deformity. The patient has been living in a wheelchair and trophic changes are seen in the dependent feet.

176 Neuralgic amyotrophy (shoulder girdle paralysis). The cause of this condition is uncertain but it is probably of viral origin, or follows immunisation serum. Following an episode of intense pain the patient has lost the ability to abduct his shoulder and there is gross wasting of the shoulder girdle musculature.

177 Simple herpes zoster skin lesion on the outer border of the foot. Prodromal or post-herpetic neuralgia may simulate 'sciatica'.

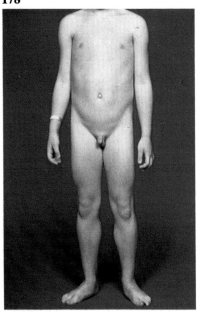

178 Progressive muscular dystrophy. This disease is transmitted by a sex-linked recessive gene. The phospho-creatinine-kinase (PCK) of the serum is raised in the patient as well as in the majority of female carriers. The child shows enlargement of the calf muscles in pseudo-hypertrophic muscular dystrophy.

179

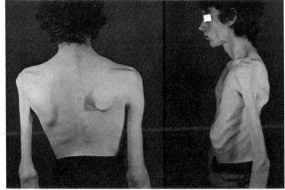

179 Progressive muscular dystrophy. The shoulder girdle and thoracic muscles become affected after a few years and the prognosis for life is poor.

180

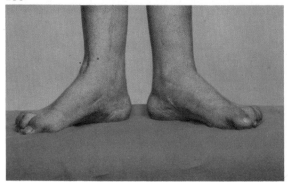

180 Pes cavus. Exaggeration of the arch of the foot is a common orthopaedic presentation of a neurological problem. A family history of high-arched foot is present in nearly half the cases of idiopathic pes cavus. It may be the only manifestation of peroneal muscular atrophy (HMSN Type I). The more carefully that any particular case of pes cavus is studied – particularly bilateral pes cavus – the more apparent becomes a neurological aetiology such as, e.g. Friedreich's disease. (see **725**)

181

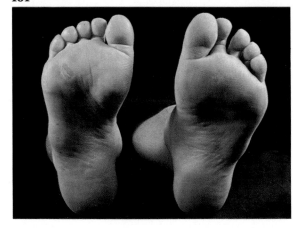

181 Progressive pes cavus: pressure points eventually develop under the heads of the metatarsals.

182

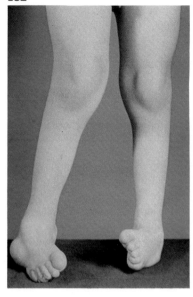

182 Peroneal muscular atrophy (Charcot-Marie-Tooth disease, HMSN Type I). Pes cavus is often the presenting symptom; shortening and distortion of the foot may, however, occur later. Wasting of the leg below the knee may be seen early in the disease. Severe talipes equino varus may develop. The gross deformity of a so-called 'Rooster's leg' is depicted here.

183

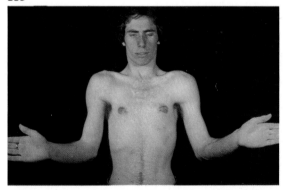

183   Wasting of the intrinsic muscles of the hands may develop late in the disease.

Facioscapulohumeral dystrophy (Déjérine myopathy)

An inheritable disorder by an autosomal dominant gene. The onset of the disease is in the second decade, after which progress is slow and relatively benign. The expectation of life is good.

184

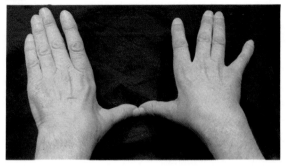

184   'Tapir mouth'. The characteristic facies with pouting lips due to weakness of orbicularis oris and oculi.

185

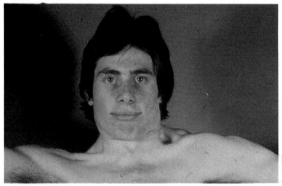

185   Note the discrepancy between the powerful arms and loss of muscle bulk of the chest.

186

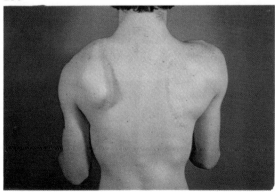

186   The right scapula has been fused to the chest wall by operation, and its stabilisation has improved shoulder girdle function on the right side.

Characteristic winging of the scapula can be seen on the unoperated left side.

Spastic paralysis

Spastic paralysis may present as an orthopaedic problem, either as a consequence of cerebral palsy in infancy, or following head injury or cerebrovascular disease.

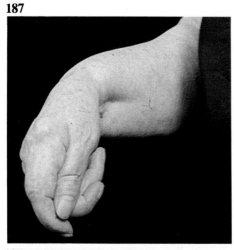

187 Cerebral palsy. Spastic contracture of the wrist and forearm, characteristically held in full flexion and pronation.

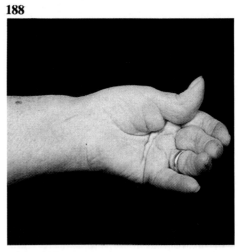

188 The thumb-in-palm position of the hand in same patient.

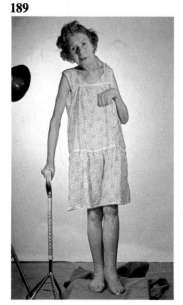

189 Hemiplegia following a cerebrovascular accident.

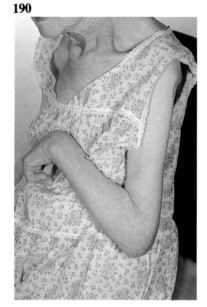

190 The upper limb is held in characteristic adduction at the shoulder, flexion at the elbow and wrist. The fingers are flexed, with thumb-in-palm position.

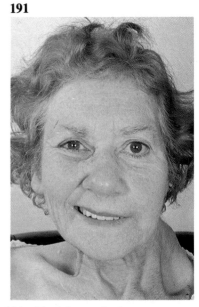

191 Facial paralysis may occur depending on the precise site of the vascular lesion.

Neuropathic arthropathy (Charcot joint)

192

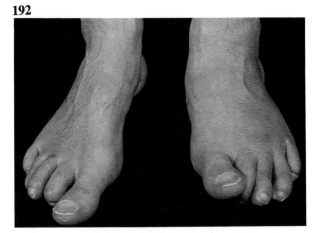

193

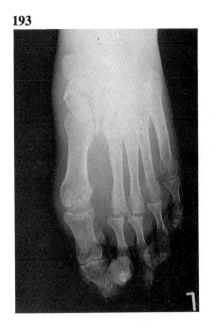

192   Diabetes. The feet of a diabetic patient with a combination of anaesthesia and peripheral vascular disease.

193   Radiographs show the disorganisation of the distal joints of the patient's foot.

194

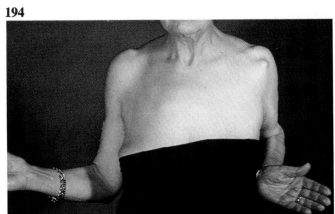

194   Syringomyelia resulting in a destructive arthropathy of the shoulder joint.

195

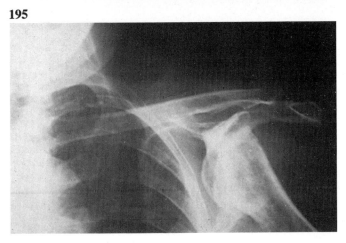

195   Radiograph of the same patient.

196

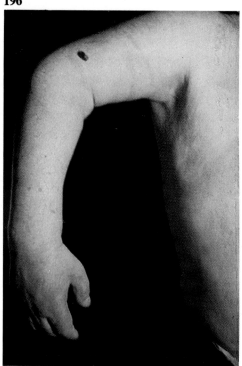

196 Syringomyelia. Flail painless elbow joint.

197

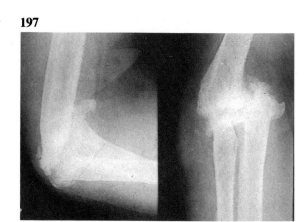

197 Radiograph of the same patient.

198

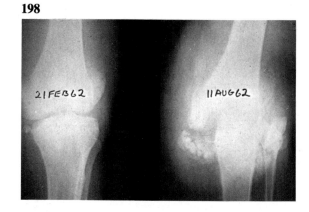

198 Tabes dorsalis. Secondary disorganisation of knee and foot joints, secondary to neurosyphilis.

199

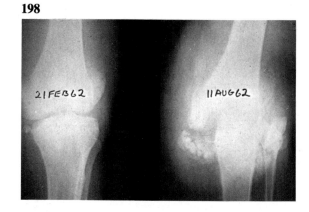

199 Radiograph of the same patient.

Hansen's disease

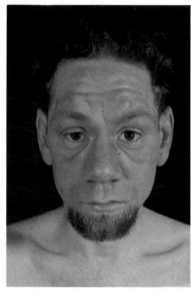

200

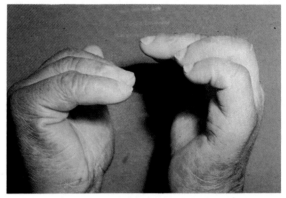

201

200 **Lepromatous leprosy.** The leonine facies.

201 Infiltration of subcutaneous tissues of the hand by granulomatous masses.

202

203

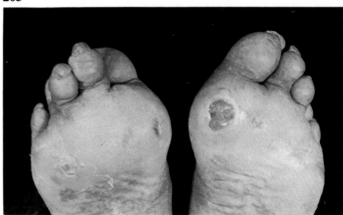

203 **Anaesthetic foot.** Trophic ulceration.

204

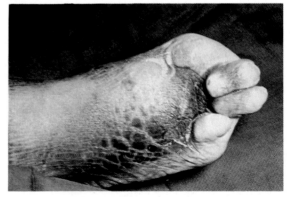

202 Intrinsic paralysis. Peripheral neuropathy leading to paralysis of the muscles of the hand and a consequent claw-hand.

204 Anaesthetic foot. Progressive absorption of anaesthetic digits due to repeated minor injury.

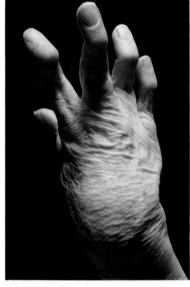

205

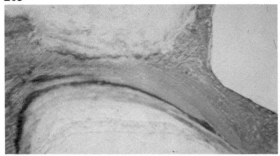

205 Normal bone. The bone salts are dyed blue; the osteoid tissue is stained pink. The relation between mature calcified bone (blue) and immature unmineralised osteoid (pink) is noted. On the righthand side of the section a resorption cavity can be seen. *(Solochrome-cyanin × 100)*

207

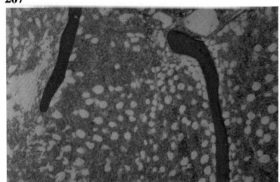

206

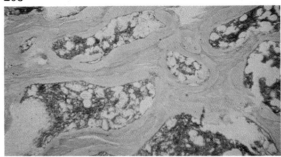

206 Osteomalacia. There is inadequate mineralisation. Decrease of mature bone (blue) compared to osteoid tissue (pink). *(× 50)*

207 Osteoporosis. The bone which has been formed is of normal composition, but there is an insufficient total amount. An undecalcified section shows that the mature bone (deep blue) is of normal structure, but considerably diminished. It lies in haemopoetic marrow.

208 Vitamin D metabolism. The stages essential to the development of normal bone. The growth and subsequent development of bone may be impaired by the interruption of vitamin D metabolism at any of the phases shown: diminished intake from skin or gut, impairment of liver function, impairment of renal function.

208

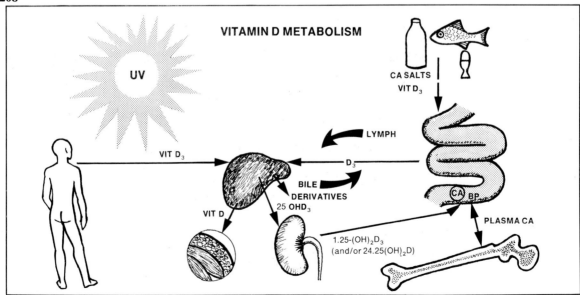

209

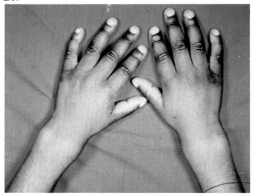

209 Nutritional rickets. The swollen wrists of a child suffering from inadequate vitamin D intake. The swelling is due to the enlargement of the radius and ulna at their lower ends where most growth occurs.

210

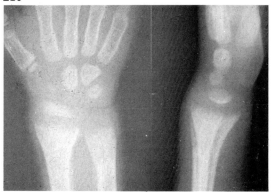

210 Radiograph to show the abnormal and enlarged growth-plates of radius and ulna due to the impairment of normal ossification of growth cartilage.

211

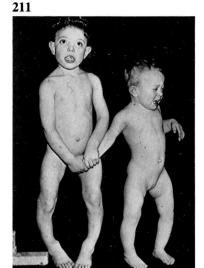

211 Hereditary hypophosphataemic rickets. In this condition the renal tubules fail to re-absorb phosphorus, thereby interfering with the normal metabolism of bone salt. One type of renal tubular deficiency rickets occurs.

212

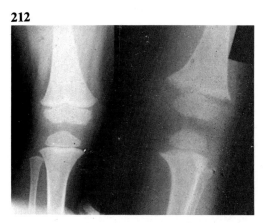

212 Rickets. Radiographs of the knee joints of a normal and rachitic child for comparison. The enlarged and irregular growth-plates and the relative loss of bone density are obvious.

213 & 214 Phenytoin rickets. This is an example of the interruption of vitamin D metabolism in the liver. Prolonged anticonvulsant therapy with phenytoin may impair vitamin D metabolism, probably by an enzyme failure in the liver. Radiographs show the severe atrophy of the distal phalanges.

213

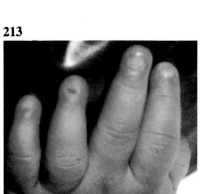

214

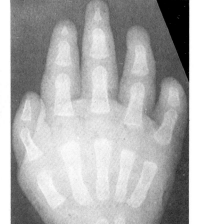

215

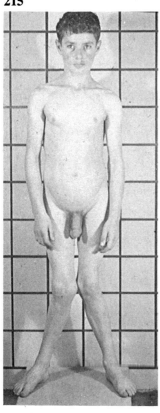

215 Rickets in a child due to renal damage. Because of impairment of renal function by kidney disease in childhood, the normal calcium-phosphorus metabolism has been altered.

216

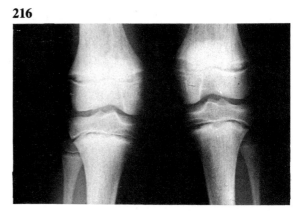

216 Radiographs of the knees in same patient.

217

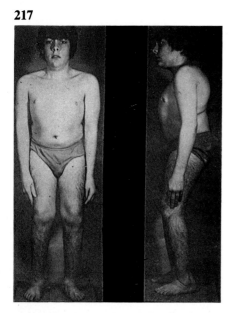

217–220 Idiopathic juvenile osteoporosis. No disturbance of vitamin D metabolism can be established and the bone which is formed is of normal density and structure, but there is too little of it. The dorsal vertebrae in this case show early collapse and a tendency to a biconcave shape.

218

219   **220**

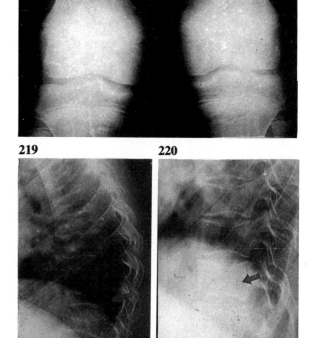

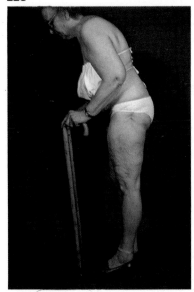

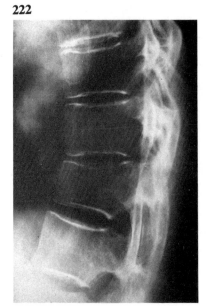

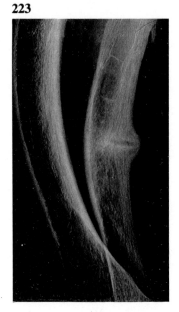

221 Senile osteoporosis. A common disorder probably related to hormonal disturbance of bone metabolism. The first clinical evidence is often the development of a simple forward spinal curvature.

222 Senile osteoporosis. Lateral radiograph of an early case.

223 A typical osteoid seam (Looser's zone) in a rib; a form of pathological fracture in osteoporosis and osteomalacia.

Parathyroid osteodystrophy

The parathyroid glands play a vital role in calcium-phosphorus metabolism and disturbance of their function is consequently noted in the skeleton. Primary hyperparathyroidism is due to a tumour of the gland and secondary hyperparathyroidism (the more common) frequently due to organic renal disease.

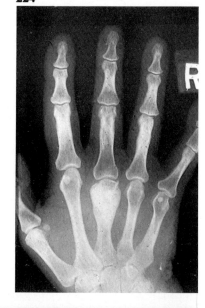

224 Primary hyperparathyroidism. Approximately 20 per cent of patients have a skeletal lesion most commonly seen in the hands. Subperiosteal resorption of the phalanges in the middle and ring fingers are noted. A 'brown tumour' expands the middle metacarpal bone.

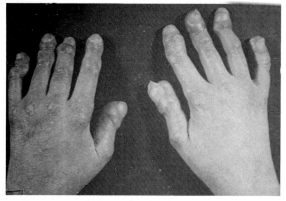

225 Secondary hyperparathyroidism to show pseudoclubbing.

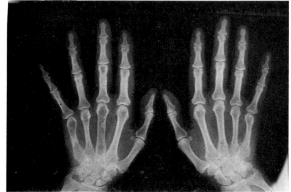

226 Radiographs show resorption of the terminal phalanges.

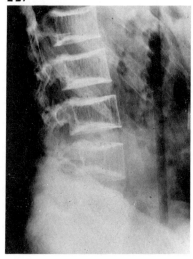

227 Typical 'rugger-jersey' effect in the spine in secondary hyperparathyroidism due to demineralisation of the vertebral bodies, with simultaneous new bone formation at the subchondral plates.

Gout

A metabolic disease of disordered metabolism of purine. Crystals of sodium urate monohydrate are deposited principally in synovial lined structures. There is a genetic linkage of clinical gout with familial hyperuricaemia.

228

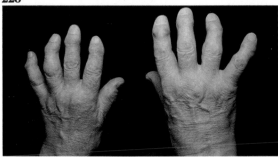

228 Repeated deposition of crystals in the joints of the fingers may ultimately lead to a destructive arthropathy.

229

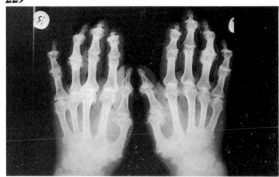

229 Radiographs of the same patient.

230

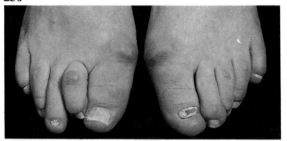

230 Classical gout presents as a bunion with a short acute history.

231

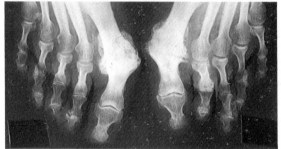

231 Typical destructive arthropathy in a long-standing case.

232

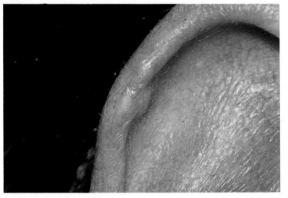

232 Gouty tophus sited in the perichondrium of the earlobe.

233

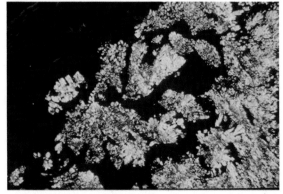

233 The crystals of sodium urate monohydrate are seen best by polarised light microscopy. *(× 400)*

Histiocytosis

A mixed group of conditions ranging from 'tumours' of cholesterol-filled cells, to widespread deposition of granulomata in bone.

234

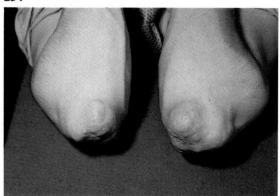

234 Simple xanthomatosis of the olecranon bursa.

235

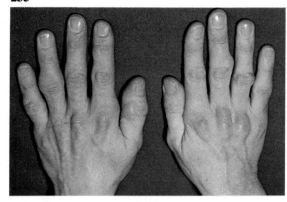

235 Hand-Schuller-Christian disease. Widespread histiocytic granulomatosis.

236

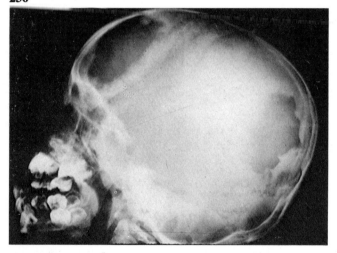

236 Radiograph of the skull in Hand-Schuller-Christian disease.

237

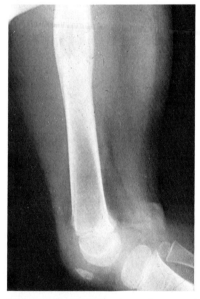

237 Eosinophilic granuloma of bone. The deposits may be single or multiple and usually recover without treatment.

238

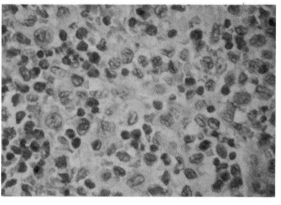

238 Eosinophilic granuloma of bone. Eosinophils dominate in the section which also contains plasma cells, lymphocytes, histiocytes and other mononuclear cells. *(× 400)*

Alkaptonuria (ochronosis)

This is a condition of autosomal recessive inheritance in which there is a defect of the metabolism of phenylalanine and tyrosine as a result of which homogentistic acid appears in the urine, which darkens on standing.

239

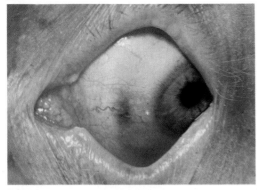

239 The sclera; dark blue melanin-like products deposited in the eyes.

240

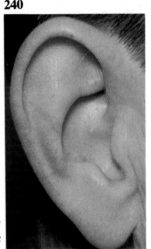

240 Ear-lobes containing deposits in the cartilage.

241

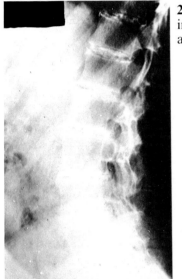

241 The intervertebral discs are affected early in ochronosis leading to a typical radiographic appearance.

242

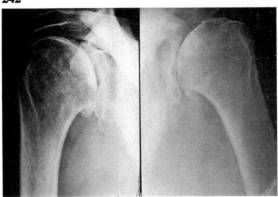

242 Ochronosis is one of the rare causes of 'osteoarthritis' of the shoulder joint; even more rarely of the hips.

243

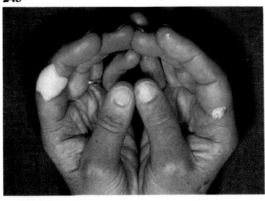

243 Calcinosis circumscripta. One of a group of collagen diseases whose clinical features are well known, but whose aetiology remains obscure. The hands are frequently affected in diffuse calcinosis.

244

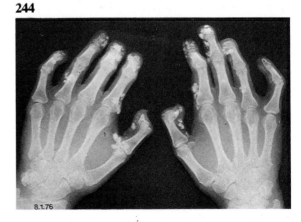

244 The radio-opaque deposits of calcium salt are easily visible on the radiographs.

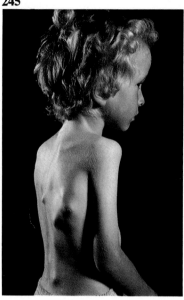

245

245 **Myositis ossificans progressive** is a rare disease in which initially painful masses appear, usually first in the cervical and shoulder girdle regions.

246

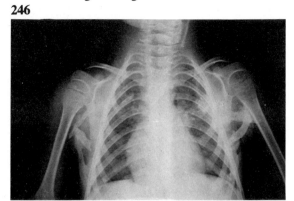

246 The masses of new bone formed in the soft tissues may restrict spine and shoulder movements as well as respiration.

Systemic sclerosis (scleroderma)

247

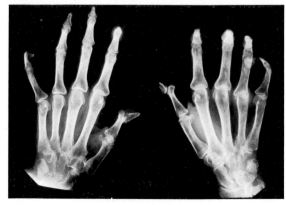

247 **Scleroderma** may involve the mouth at an early stage. Patients develop pinched mask-like facies.

248

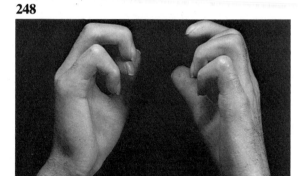

248 **Scleroderma.** Hands of a patient to show taut shiny skin extending to involve all the joints with some atrophy of the distal segments of the fingers.

249

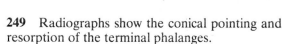

249 Radiographs show the conical pointing and resorption of the terminal phalanges.

250 **Systemic sclerosis:** the skin of the feet is typically shiny, taut and atrophic.

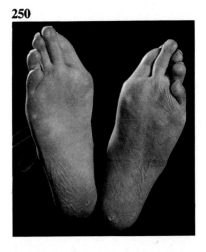

250

Mucopolysaccharide disorders

This is a group of occasionally serious skeletal disorders, characterised by an inborn error of the metabolism of mucopolysaccharide (MPS). The group is very variable but they all have the metabolic disorder in common. The best known is Morquio-Brailsford disease (MPS IV), with characteristic involvement of spine and hip joints. Dwarfing is due to the short trunk. There is no mental retardation. The condition is of autosomal recessive inheritance.

251

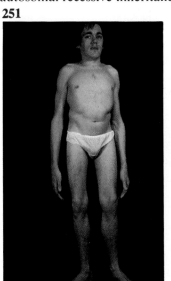

252

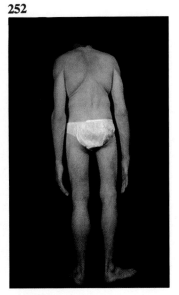

253

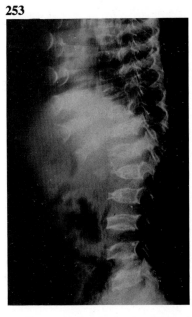

251 & 252   Morquio-Brailsford disease showing the characteristic short trunk with normal length of arms. The head is typically set into the thorax due to an increase in the manubriosternal angle which is a right-angle or more.

253   The typical anterior beaking of the lower dorsal and upper lumbar vertebrae.

254

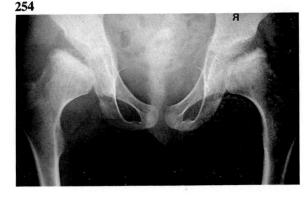

254   Bilateral flattening and irregularity of the femoral heads, resembling severe Perthes' disease.

Paget's disease of bone

This is a disease of unknown origin which mainly affects the skeletal system of middle-aged and elderly people, and is most common in Great Britain, United States and Australasia. Night pain, deformity, progressive enlargement of the head, bone deafness and other complications may occur. There are three phases: destructive; bone forming; and combined.

255

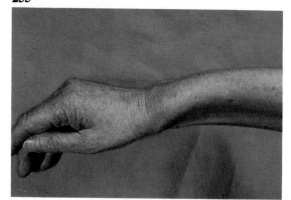

256

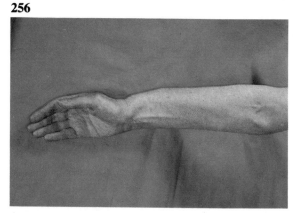

255 & 256   Deformity of the forearm due to enlargement and elongation of the radius.

257

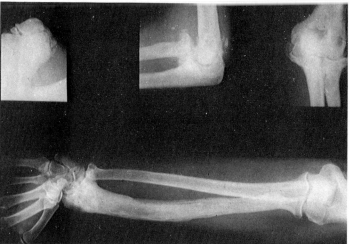

257   A skeletal survey showed that the opposite elbow joint was also affected.

258

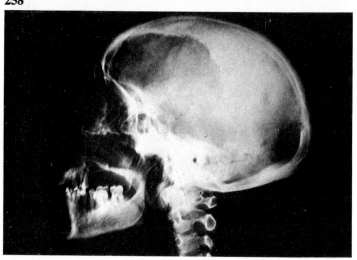

258   The skull showed typical changes of the acute phase of Paget's disease, known as osteoporosis circumscripta.

259–262 **Paget's disease of bone** in its more advanced stage. The patient has a 'sabre' tibia due to actual enlargement of length and bulk of the tibia with anterior bowing. Almost the entire skeleton was involved. The skull shows a more advanced stage of the disease with new bone accretion on the cortex.

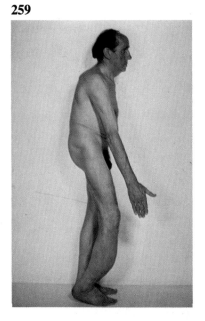

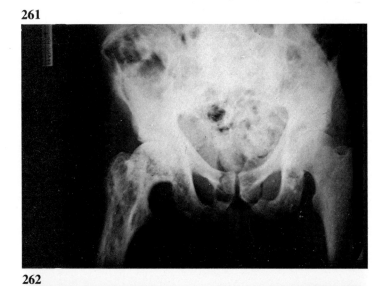

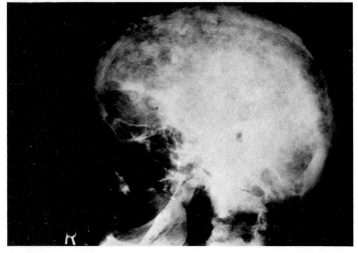

263

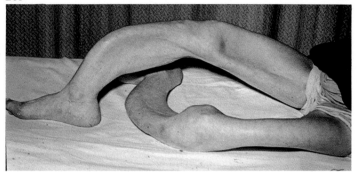

264

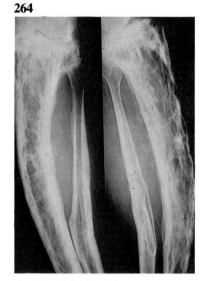

263 & 264 Advanced form of Paget's disease with gross bowing of the tibia and alteration of architectural pattern. The alkaline phosphatase of this patient was raised to between 65 and 100 Ka units (about 10 units is normal).

265

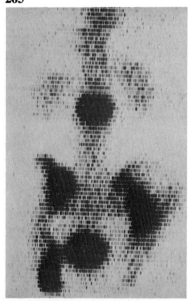

265 Radio-isotope scanning shows considerable increase of uptake of the bone-seeking isotope technetium by the most affected parts of the skeleton.

266

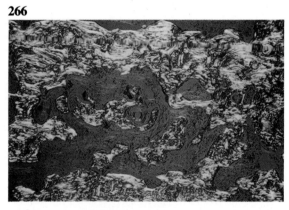

266 Non-lamellar arrangement (woven) bone in Paget's disease viewed in polarised light. *(× 75)*

267

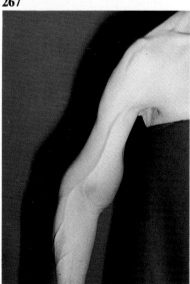

267 Paget's sarcoma of the humerus. Approximately 1 per cent of cases of Paget's disease may advance to develop a sarcoma of variable cell type.

268

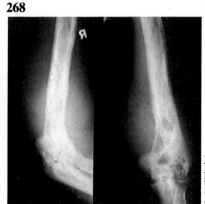

268 Radiograph of the same patient. Note the soft tissue swelling, as well as destruction of the medial cortex.

Fibrous dysplasia of bone

There are three forms of fibrous dysplasia of bone, a disease of unknown origin which usually presents in the first two decades of life.

269

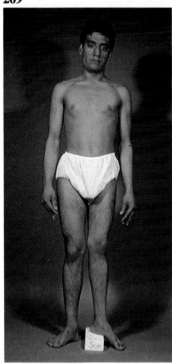

269 Monostotic fibrous dysplasia affecting the femur in a 20-year-old man.

270

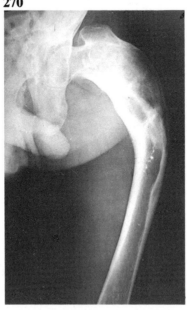

270 The condition was symptomless until a pathological fracture occurred and healed with bowing.

271

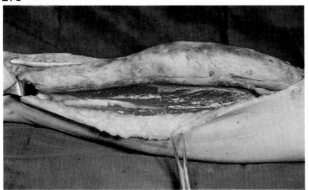

271 The enlarged and distorted femoral shaft seen at operation. The medullary bone had been replaced by fibrous tissues.

272

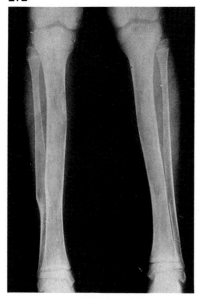

273

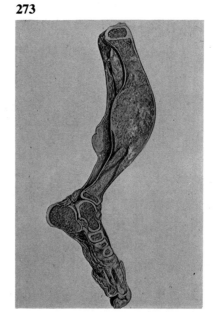

272 Polyostotic fibrous dysplasia. There is a widespread distribution of lesions without systemic disturbance.

273 Fibrous dysplasia in a tibia.

274

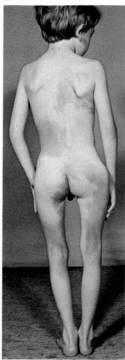

275

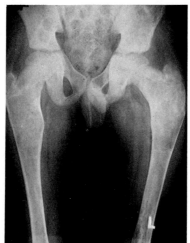

275 Fibrotic areas in the bone appear as scattered patches of rarefaction. The lesions are predominantly unilateral. The epiphyses are not affected. The lower extremities are most frequently and extensively involved.

274 Albright's syndrome. Polyostotic fibrous dysplasia associated with cutaneous pigmentation and sexual precocity (usually female).

Benign tumours of soft-tissue, cartilage and bone

276

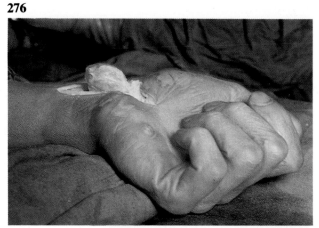

276   Ganglion. The commonest tumour seen in orthopaedic practice consists of a simple pseudo-cyst containing viscous fluid. It usually arises from the synovial membrane of a joint or tendon sheath. The ganglion here depicted originated in the sheath of flexor carpi ulnaris.

277

277   Simple ganglion arising from the ankle joint.

278

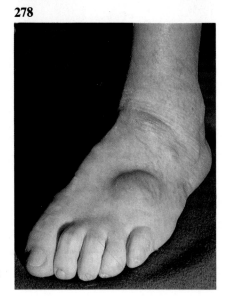

278   Lipoma in the subcutaneous fat on the dorsum of the foot.

279 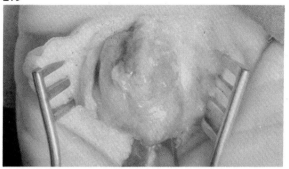 **280**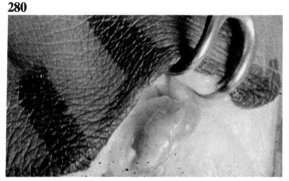

279 Pigmented villonodular synovitis. This is a non-malignant but locally invasive condition arising from synovial membrane. It is commonest in the knee joint but is also seen in wrist, hand and other joints.

280 & 281 PVNS of the metacarpo-phalangeal joint of the ring finger extending through from palmar to dorsal surfaces. Careful inspection of the radiograph shows typical erosion of the base of the proximal phalanx of the affected joint.

281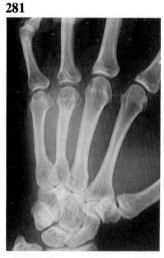

282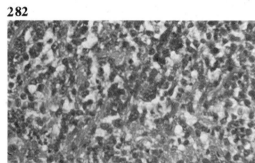

282 A mixed inflammatory cell infiltrate in which multinucleated giant cells are present scattered throughout the fibrofatty connective tissue. Tiny fragments of iron-staining material are evident. (× 200)

283 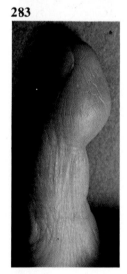 **284** 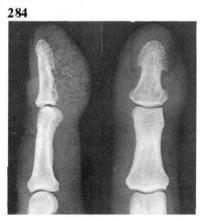 **285**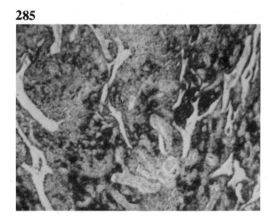

285 Perl stained for iron pigment; the lesion is more mature and the collagen tissue is more dense. (× 50)

283–284 PVNS in the pulp of an index finger probably arising from the terminal IP joint.

286

287

288

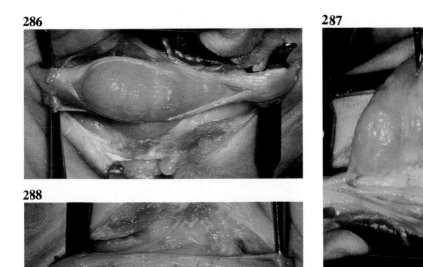

286–288 **Intraneural lipoma** is shelled out of the ulnar nerve at the wrist. It lies within the nerve sheath but does not penetrate the nerve bundles, which remain intact after removal.

289

290

291

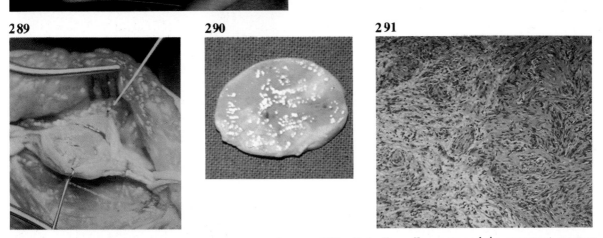

289 & 290 **Neurilemmoma (Schwannoma).** An innocent tumour arising from the Schwann cells of peripheral nerve and only very gradually affecting the nerve-conducting tissues by direct pressure. There is no infiltration so that the tumour can be shelled out without damaging the nerve fibres.

291 **Spindle cells** arranged in compact groups separated by loose areolar tissue (Antoni type A and type B tissues). *(× 85)*

292

293

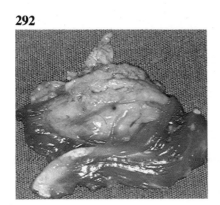

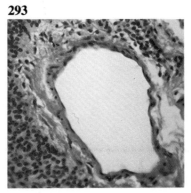

292 **Glomus tumour.** A rare but very painful tiny tumour, characteristically found in fingers and toes, sometimes beneath the nail. The tissue shown is about 5cm in diameter, but the tumour itself is only the very central portion of this, and is minute.

293 Round to oval cells of considerable uniformity surrounding a blood vessel. *(× 200)*

Congenital vascular malformation

294

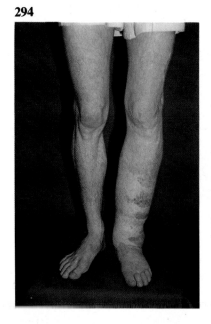

295

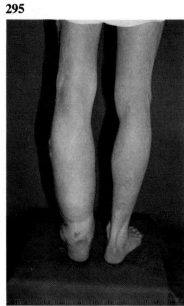

294 & 295 A network of veins and capillaries extending through the muscles, subcutaneous tissue and skin of most of the left leg. The increase in girth and the discolouration of the skin are evident. There was no increase in length in this case.

296

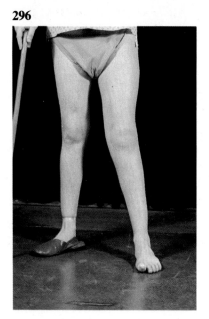

297

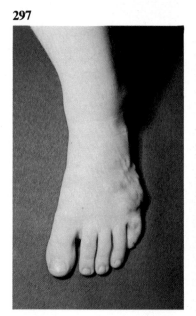

298

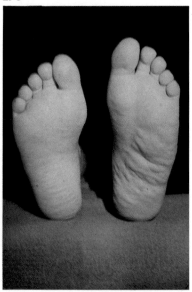

296–8 Congenital arteriovenous malformation affecting the whole of the left lower limb in a young man. In the thigh it was contained within the substance of the quadriceps muscle and in the foot it was evident on the dorsal and plantar surfaces. In addition to local swelling and obvious vascular malformation there was an increase in girth and length of the limb.

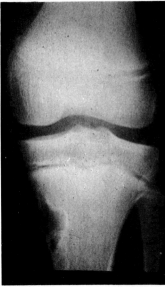

299 Non-osteogenic fibroma of bone: an incidental finding on a radiograph. This is possibly the only lesion of bone which can be diagnosed with certainty by radiographs alone. It is entirely benign.

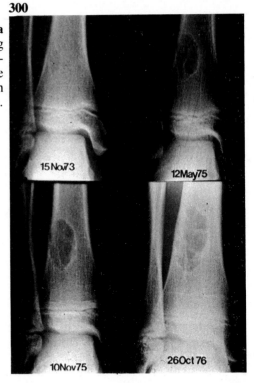

300 Non-osteogenic fibroma at the lower end of the tibia. Within three years the lesion has altered in shape and size and is beginning to fade.

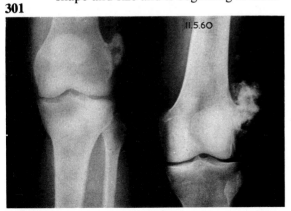

301 Osteochondroma ('exostosis'). A mass is seen arising from the lower end of the femur pointing away from the growth-plate.

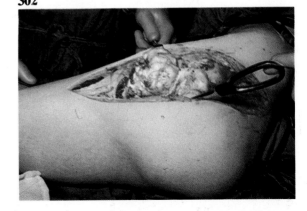

302 The osteochondroma is displayed at operation when its cartilage cap is clearly noted.

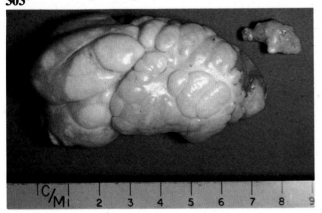

303 The resected osteochondroma.

Osteoid osteoma

This little tumour causes intense and characteristic pain and is often difficult to locate.

304

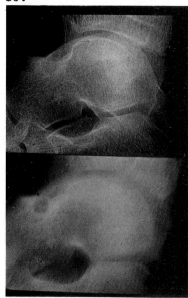

304   A typical osteoid osteoma in the neck of the talus. In the plain film above it is barely visible; in the tomograph below the characteristic nidus surrounded by a transparent moat is clearly visible.

305

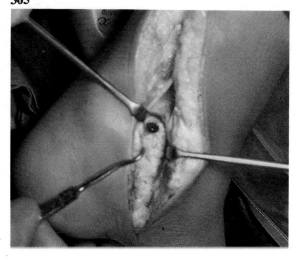

305   The pink soft tumour seen at operation.

306

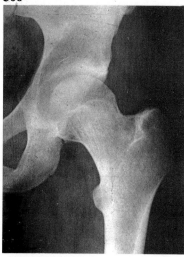

307

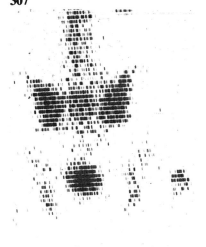

306   Osteoid osteoma at the base of the greater trochanter, only visualised with difficulty in the plain radiographs.

307   The bone scan shows a marked increase of uptake of radioactive technetium in the region of the greater trochanter.

308

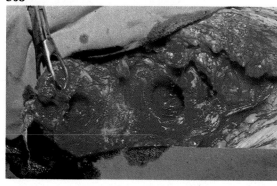

308   When the trochanter is lifted at operation the nidus containing the soft tumour is clearly visible.

309

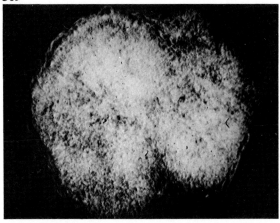

309　A slab radiograph of the material removed from **308**. The whole lesion has been lifted from its bed in the bone and in the centre of the cancellous bone lies a small soft mass.

310

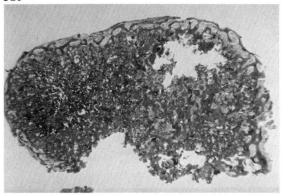

310　The tumour is composed of short irregular immature bone trabeculae in vascular fibrous tissue which contains some osteoclasts. (× 5)

Benign osteoblastoma

This is also classified as a 'giant osteoid osteoma' because it has many of the same characteristics except for its size.

311

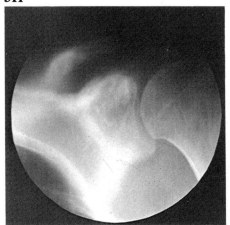

311　Pain in the shoulder region and loss of normal shoulder movements were the presenting features. Plain radiographs appeared normal, but tomography revealed a lesion in the neck of the scapula.

312

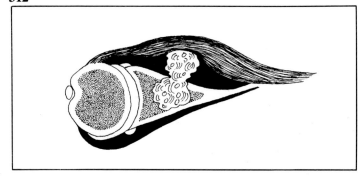

312　A diagram of the tumour as seen at operation. It arises from the neck of the scapula and bulges out backwards to lift the belly of supraspinatus muscle. This relation accounted for the fact that the patient was unable normally to abduct his shoulder prior to operation.

313

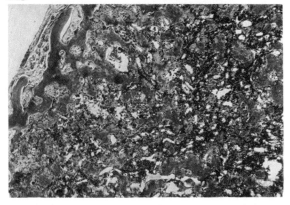

313　The lesion showing the same characteristics as osteoid osteoma. (× 100)

Haemangioma of bone

Although this condition is innocent in the sense that it does not metastasize, it may be locally extremely destructive. It varies from a single relatively simple lesion, e.g. of a vertebral body, to an extensive destructive lesion of a long bone. An extreme example, as is depicted here, is of the 'vanishing bone syndrome' of Gorham.

314

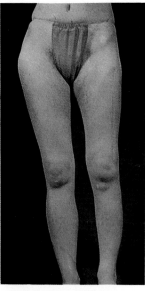

314 A 24-year-old girl with swelling, pain and deformity in the upper end of the right femur.

315

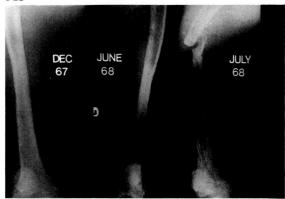

315 Serial radiographs of the femur. In the course of eight months the lesion has advanced very rapidly and a pathological fracture finally occurred.

316

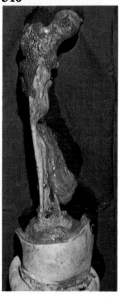

316 The specimen is resected for replacement by a prosthesis.

317

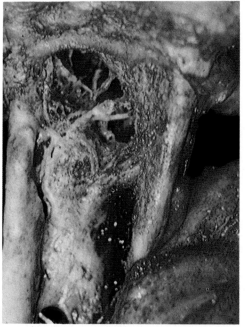

317 Enlargement of the specimen to show the considerable resorption of the osseous trabeculae, the remainder being very thickened and running vertically. The characteristic 'sunburst' reticulated appearance is well-shown.

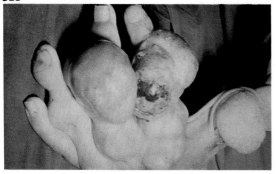

318

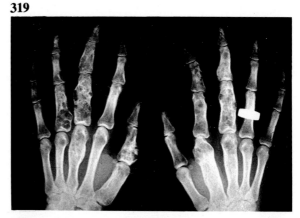

319

318 & 319 Maffucci's syndrome. An extreme form of enchondromatosis associated with hae-mangiomata in soft tissue.

320

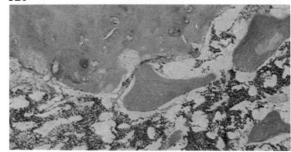

320 One of the cartilage tumours: sheets of benign cartilage cells lie above and normal marrow lies below. *(× 85)*

Aneurysmal bone cyst

This is a tumour-like lesion within bone consisting of a cavity filled with blood. The lesion expands, thins and destroys the cortex. It is benign.

321

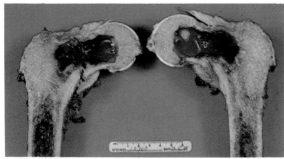

321 Aneurysmal bone cyst occupying the neck of a femur through which a pathological fracture has occurred.

322

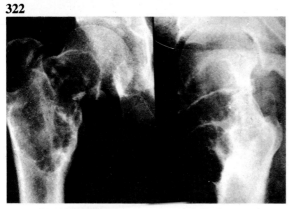

322 An aneurysmal bone cyst in a similar position.

323

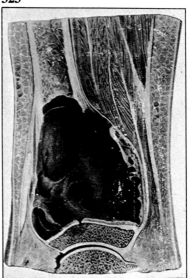

323 Pathological specimen of an aneurysmal bone cyst at the lower end of the tibia.

Giant cell tumour (osteoclastoma)

These tumours occupy a position between benign and malignant tumours. About 40 per cent of the tumours are entirely benign, about 40 per cent are locally invasive and recurrent, and the remainder metastasize.

324

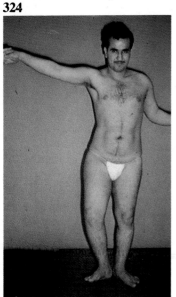

325

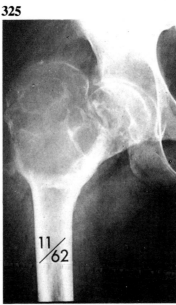

326

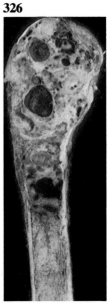

324 & 325   Giant cell tumour at the upper end of the right femur causing pain and deformity. The radiograph shows that a pathological fracture has probably occurred. The tumour usually originates at the end of a long bone and is commonest around the knee joint. The cortex is expanded and the bone is honeycombed. It extends to and involves the sub-cortical bone.

326   **The lacunae** contain solid tumour material in this pathological specimen.

327

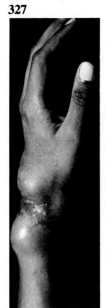

327   An advanced giant cell tumour of the lower end of the radius. The waist of the dumb-bell shaped tumour is due to the extensor retinaculum.

328

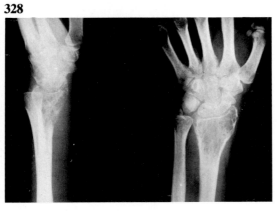

328   Radiograph of the tumour.

329

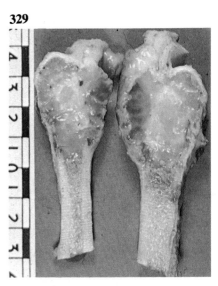

329   The specimen removed at operation.

330

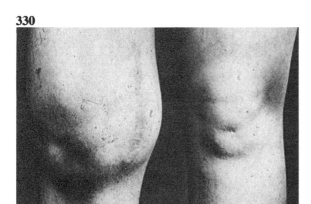

331

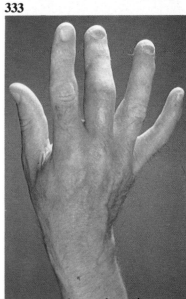

330 Giant cell tumour in its typical site at the lower end of the femur which has recurred after surgical currettage.

331 Radiograph of the tumour, typically abutting against the articular surface.

332

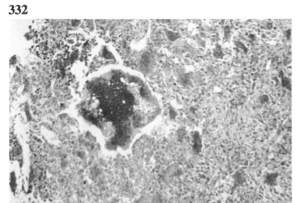

332 In a stroma of round and oval cells, there are numerous small multinucleated cells of varying size. *(× 200)*

334

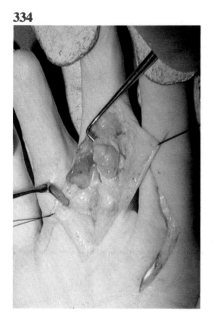

333

333 A giant cell tumour – almost always innocent – occasionally arises from synovial tendon sheath. It has developed in the flexor tendon sheath of the right middle finger.

334 The tumour displayed at operation.

Primary malignant tumours of soft tissues

335

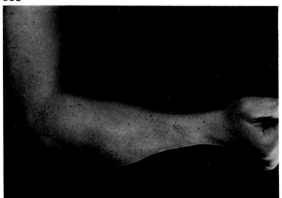

335 Fibrosarcoma. A mass in the forearm of a young man which was solid and attached to deep structures but not to skin.

336

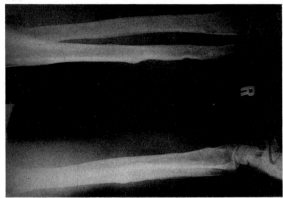

336 The ulna has become eroded from without.

337

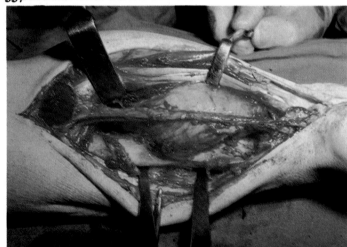

337 The tumour mass displayed at operation.

338

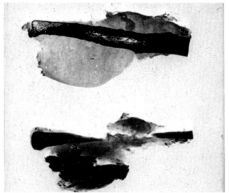

338 A slab radiograph of the resected ulna.

339

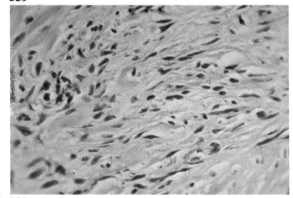

339 Bundles of fibroblasts interspersed by collagen. *(× 350)*

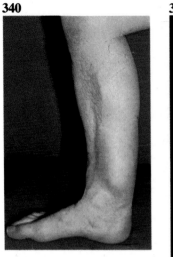

340

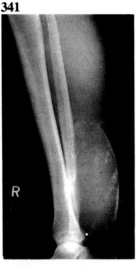

341

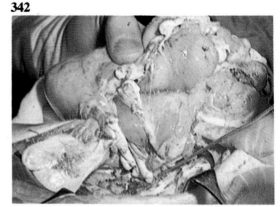

342

342 The large tumorous mass is excised.

340 & 341 Myxosarcoma. A solid mass arising in the postero-medial aspect of the lower half of the right leg of a middle-aged man. Radiograph showing an apparently encapsulated soft tissue mass with specks of calcification and new bone formation.

343 The tumour has many unusual features. It is composed of stellate myxoid cells with pools of mucin. It was considered to be a myxosarcoma. The patient died of pulmonary metastases three years later. (× 200)

343

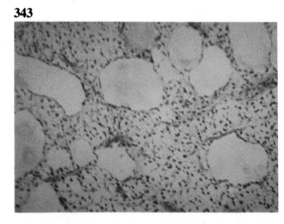

344

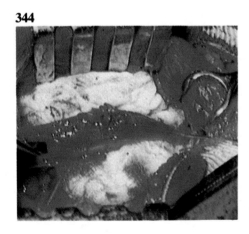

345

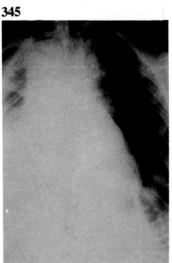

346

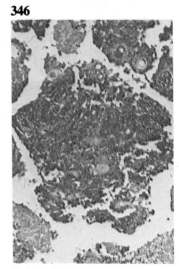

344 Malignant tumour of the sciatic nerve. This patient presented with one simple symptom: when the back of his thigh was pressed upon he experienced tingling in his big toe! There were absolutely no other abnormal symptoms or signs. At operation a fatty tumour was found to lie within the substance of the sciatic nerve in the upper third of the thigh, and extended intra-neurally upwards.

345 The patient died eighteen years later of massive mediastinal secondary deposits.

346 The tumour had the same appearances at the primary and secondary sites. The cellular tumour showed extensive areas of necrosis. It is an undifferentiated malignant neoplasm located within a nerve, classified as a neurosarcoma. (× 100)

347

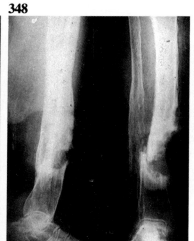

348

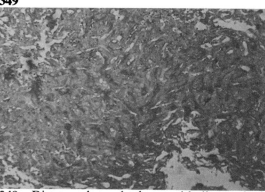

349

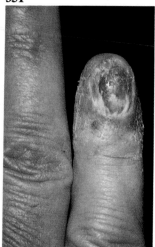

349 Biopsy showed that epithelioma had developed in the Yaws ulcer. The leg was amputated.

348 The tibia has been eroded by the soft tissue disease surrounding it.

347 Diagnosed as Yaws. This patient had an ulcer on the medial aspect of her right lower leg for many years. A sudden increase in the extent of the ulcerated area and the increase of pain caused her to seek medical advice.

351

350

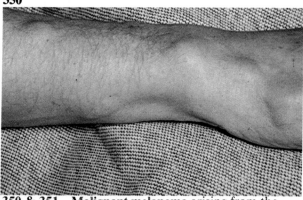

350 & 351 Malignant melanoma arising from the nail-bed of the little finger. The malignant melanoma has spread along the lymphatics and a secondary tumour has developed on the dorsum of the lower forearm.

Chondrosarcoma

352 Chondrosarcoma of the upper end of the femur, which has enlarged and distorted the bone.

353

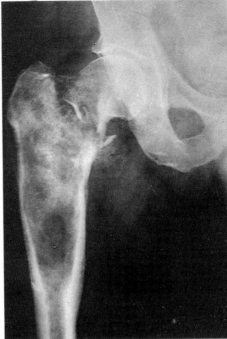

352

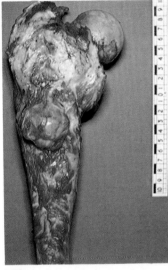

353 Radiograph showing that a pathological fracture has occurred at the base of the neck of the femur.

354

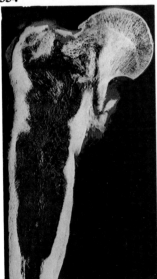

355

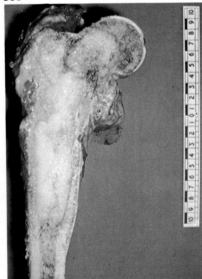

356

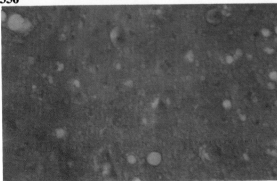

354 Slab radiograph of the specimen which delineates its extent and also confirms the pathological fracture.

355 Hemisection of the specimen to show tumour cartilage occupying and expanding the bone.

356 The specimen shows a mass of immature cartilage cells with multiple mitotic figures. *(× 400)*

Osteosarcoma

357
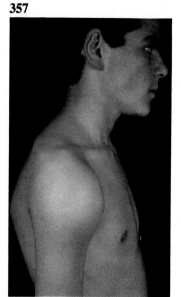

358
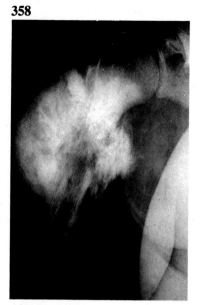

357 A large painful swelling in a fifteen-year-old boy at the proximal end of the right humerus. It had appeared in only a few weeks. At least half of the cases of osteosarcoma are situated around the knee joint but any bone may be affected. It can simulate osteomyelitis.

358 Radiograph shows the lytic defects within the bone, periosteal new bone formation, and the characteristic 'sunray' spiculation.

359
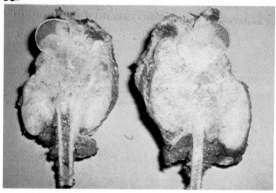

359 The specimen removed by disarticulation at the shoulder.

Ewing's tumour

360
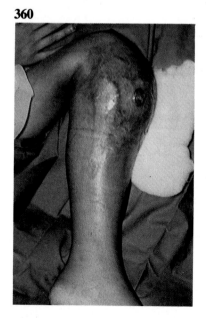

361
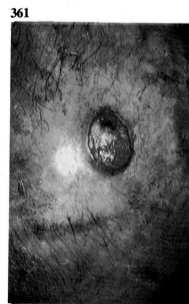

360 Ewing's tumour: an advanced case of the upper end of the tibia in a teenage boy, which has not responded to radiotherapy. Severe pain and constitutional disturbances are a feature.

361 The centre of the tumour has ulcerated through the skin. Dilated veins are seen in the lower half of the tumour.

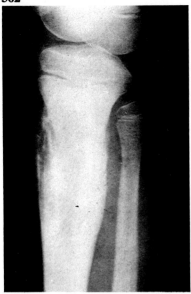

362 Radiograph of the tumour shows a mottled destructive pattern, without any clear zone of transition, involving the medulla of the bone and permeating the anterior cortex.

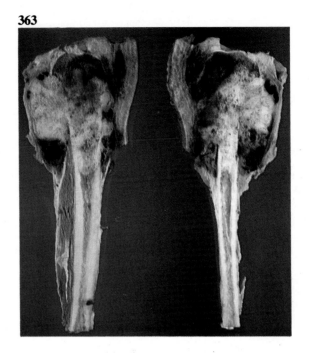

363 Tumour specimen recovered at amputation.

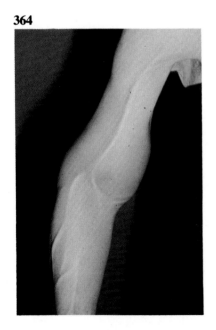

364 **Paget's sarcoma** of the humerus (see **267 & 268**).

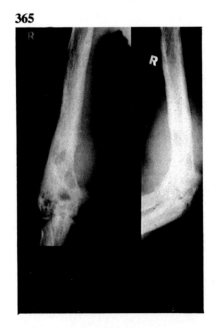

365 The radiograph appearances are characterised by a destructive type of lesion with relatively irregular new bone formation.

Secondary malignant tumours of bone

Secondary malignant tumours of the skeleton are very much more common than primary malignant tumours. The typical primary sites from which secondary deposits occur are bronchus, kidney, breast, thyroid, large intestine and prostate. A few examples are shown here.

366

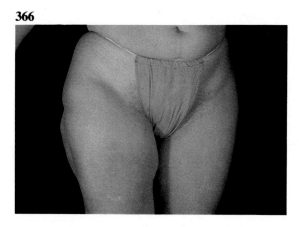

366 Thyroid. This 52-year-old lady had pain and swelling in the upper aspect of her right thigh. Two years previously a malignant adenoma had been removed from her thyroid.

367

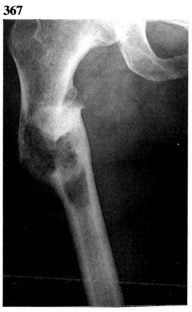

367 An isolated translucent deposit with very little bone reaction is seen: a pathological fracture has occurred through the malignant secondary deposit from the primary in the thyroid gland.

368

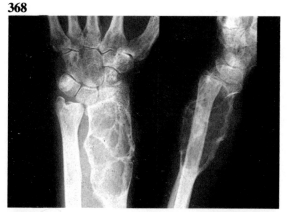

369

368 Kidney. Enlarged lower end of radius. There was increased warmth of the overlying skin and a vascular bruit could be heard. The honeycombed appearance of the expanded lower end of radius with considerable thinning of the cortex is noted. The appearances are characteristic of a secondary hypernephroma.

369 The primary tumour in the right kidney is confirmed by pyelography.

370

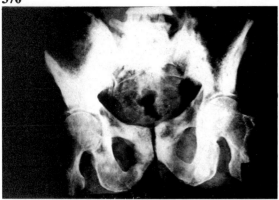

370 Prostate. Carcinoma of the prostate may produce widespread skeletal deposits which have a characteristically dense osteoblastic appearance.

371

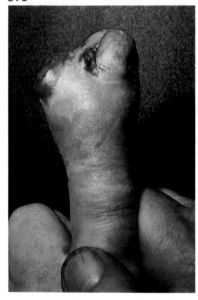

372

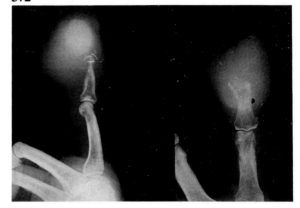

372   Radiograph of the tumour.

371 Rectum. An ulcerated tumour of the enlarged tip of an index finger due to secondary carcinoma. The primary was in the rectum.

Regional section

Most orthopaedic problems present as a disorder of some localised part of the body, usually a joint. Having satisfied oneself that the presenting feature is not an expression of generalised musculo-skeletal disease, one can confidently proceed to a detailed clinical study of the local lesion. In the pages which follow some examples are presented of localised physical disorders commonly met with in clinical orthopaedic practice.

373

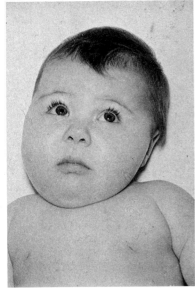

373 Torticollis (Wry neck). The sternomastoid muscle on the left side of this child's neck is contracted so that his head is tilted to the left and rotated to the right. In 20 per cent of cases a transient 'sternomastoid tumour' can be felt in the affected muscle.

374

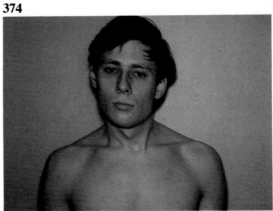

374 The deformity may persist into adult life. The tilting and rotation of the head become established and the eyes remain at different levels. The prominent manubrial head of the left sternomastoid muscle is clearly shown.

375

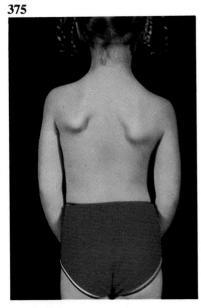

375 Sprengel's shoulder. This child's left scapula has failed to descend from its embryonic position.

376

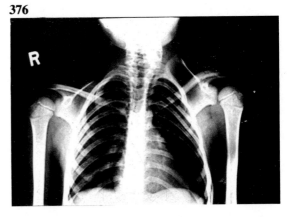

376 Radiograph to show the high, cervical position of the scapula.

377

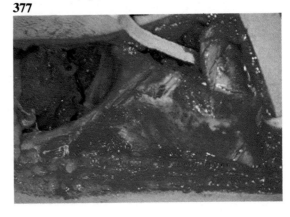

377 A fibrous band extends between the upper border of the scapula and the cervical vertebrae. This band may become ossified (omovertebral bone). The band is displayed at operation by the upper retractor.

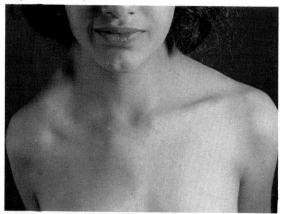

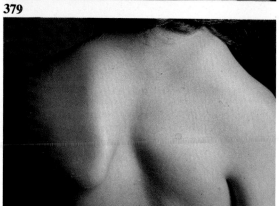

378 & 379 Klippel-Feil syndrome. There is a bilateral failure of scapular descent usually associated with considerable abnormality of the cervical vertebrae. The neck is very short and webbed, with a low hairline.

380 The radiograph shows scoliosis with a jumble of unsegmented cervical vertebrae.

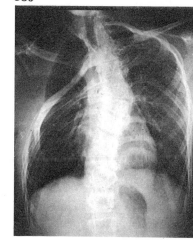

Cervical spondylosis

381 Degenerative arthritis of the cervical spine is such a common condition as to be considered as a normal feature of biological ageing. The fact that cervical spondylosis is demonstrated on a radiograph does not necessarily indicate a disease process responsible for the patient's symptoms. The histograph shows how commonly radiographic cervical spondylosis appears in the general population.

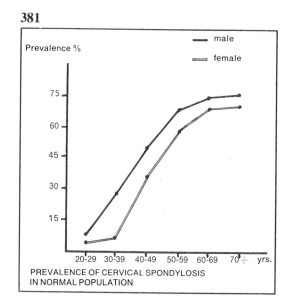

PREVALENCE OF CERVICAL SPONDYLOSIS
IN NORMAL POPULATION

382

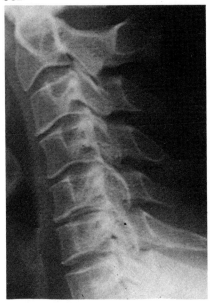

382 Acute cervical intervertebral disc protrusion. Often the only abnormality seen is the loss of normal cervical lordosis in the lateral radiographs. It is due to muscle spasm. The bone and joint structure may be otherwise entirely normal in early cases.

383 **384**

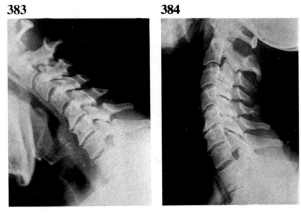

383 & 384 Radiographs of the cervical spine taken in full flexion and extension showing marked spondylosis at the commonest level, C5/6, symptomless in this case.

385

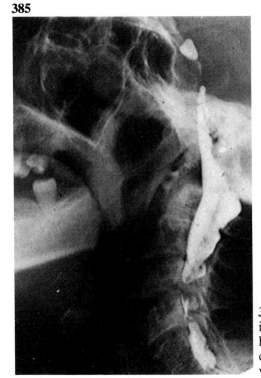

385 Cervical myelography. Interruption of the myodil column, rarely caused by the pressure of osteophytes and disc material in cervical spondylosis.

386

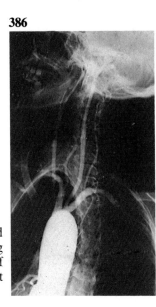

386 Angiography. Unexplained intermittent syncope. On turning her head to the left, the flow of contrast medium through the left vertebral artery is interrupted.

Thoracic outlet (cervical rib) syndrome

387

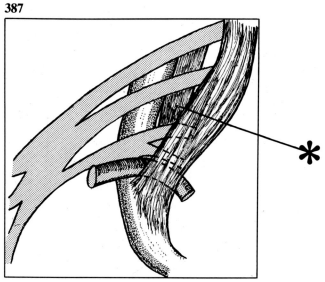

387 The subclavian artery and the lower trunk of the brachial plexus (C8, T1) lie – as it were – suspended in a sling formed by scalenus anticus insertion in front and the first rib behind. An extra rib arising from C8, its fibrous equivalent, or an abnormal scalenus medius muscle, can sharpen the angle and embarrass nerve and artery. The asterisk marks the position of such an anomalous structure.

388 **389**

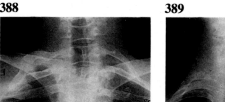 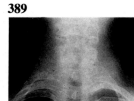

388 & 389 Bilateral cervical ribs. On the left the standard projection just shows the abnormal ribs; on the right a tilted projection of the same patient displays the ribs more clearly.

390

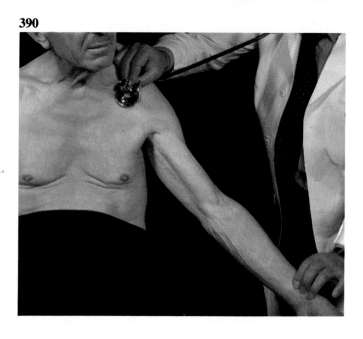

390 Adson's test. The patient's arm is pulled upon whilst his head turns towards and tilts away from, the affected side. The earliest sign of a thoracic outlet syndrome may be partial obliteration of the subclavian artery giving rise to a bruit and diminution or obliteration of the radial pulse.

391 The cervical sympathetic nerve fibres are concentrated in the lower part of the trunk of T1. Irritation of these fibres by a cervical rib or abnormal band may cause blanching of the skin of the hand and fingers.

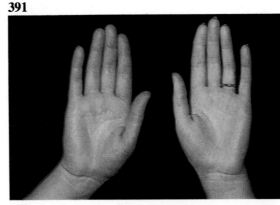

392 At a later stage, interruption of conduction of the fibres of T1 may cause wasting of the intrinsic muscles of the hand. The hypothenar muscles are shown here to be severely wasted.

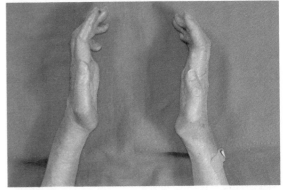

393 Occasionally no cervical rib is seen in the radiographs but an elongation of the transverse processes of the lowest cervical vertebra is noted. Probably a fibrous band extends from the tips of these to the first or second ribs.

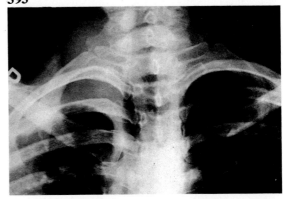

394 A well-developed fibrous band seen at operation in the position of scalenus medius lying behind the first thoracic nerve root and impairing its normal conduction.

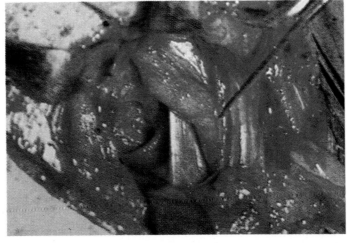

Dorsal spine

395

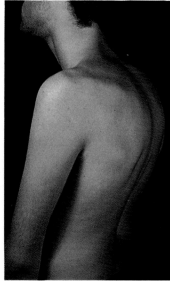

396

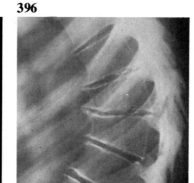

395 & 396 Adolescent Kyphosis (Scheurmann's disease). An adolescent becomes 'round-shouldered', and he may or may not have accompanying pain in the early stages. The curve is rigid and not correctable. Several segments of the spine are involved so that the angle is not an acute one, i.e. it is a long-segment kyphosis. There is no disturbance of general health.

397

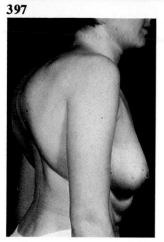

398

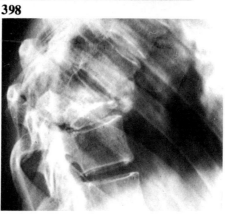

399

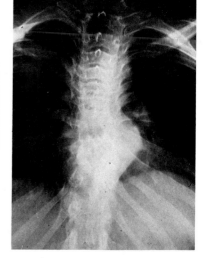

397 Tuberculosis of the spine (Pott's disease). Apart from the general disturbance of health, local pain, abscess formation and other important complications, the curve itself is distinguished by its more acute angle, due to the fact that only one or two vertebrae are usually involved. It is a short-segment kyphosis. The lateral radiograph (**398**) shows that the infection in the spine probably started between two midthoracic vertebrae and that the lower one has almost completely collapsed. The anteroposterior radiograph (**399**) shows a left-sided paravertebral abscess.

400

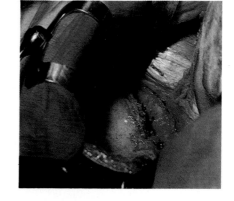

400 The abscess displayed immediately to the left of the thoracic aorta at operation.

Spina bifida

Spina bifida is caused by the failure of the two halves of the neural arch to fuse in foetal development. In Great Britain its incidence is approximately 3 per 1 000 live births. It varies in severity from a simple incidental finding on a radiograph to protrusion of elements of the spinal cord with complete paralysis below the level of the lesion. Some examples are given here.

401

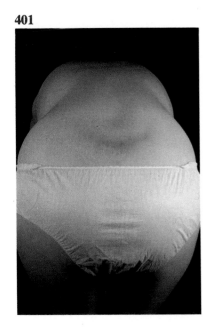

402

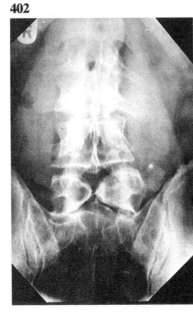

401 Fine cutaneous capillaries and slight depression over the lower part of the lumbar region of the spine. Occasionally there may be tufts of hair.

402 The radiograph shows that the 5th lumbar and 1st sacral vertebrae have failed to fuse posteriorly in the midline.

403

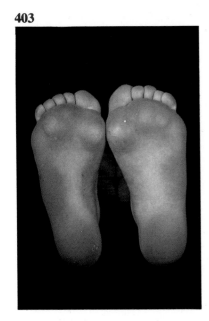

403 Pes cavus (from **401**) due to muscle imbalance.

404

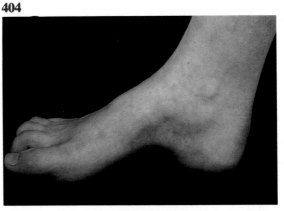

404 The pes cavus is usually accompanied by slight clawing of the toes.

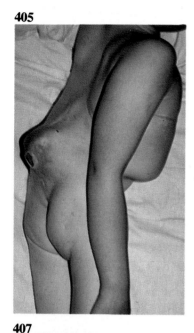

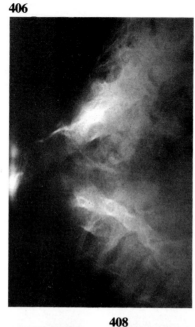

405 **A more severe form of spina bifida,** closed at birth, but the attenuated overlying tissues began to ulcerate converting it into an open type of spina bifida. There was complete spastic paralysis from the waist downwards.

406 Radiographs show the gross kyphosis at the site of extensive failure of fusion in the dorsilumbar segments.

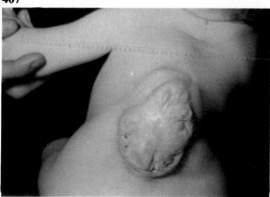

407 **Open spina bifida.** Elements of the meninges and surrounding fat covering the spinal cord are exposed.

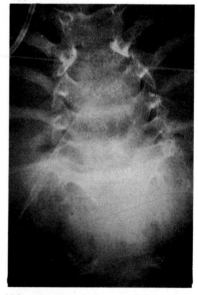

408 Radiograph to show extensive failure of fusion of the midlumbar segments.

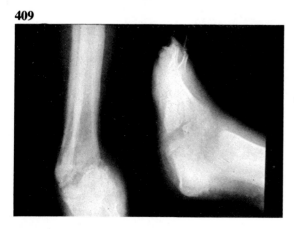

409 **Neuropathic arthropathy (Charcot's joints)** in the same child resulting in disorganisation of the ankle and hindfoot.

Scoliosis

Broadly speaking, scoliosis (spinal curvature) is either mobile or fixed. The mobile variety may be seen as a transient postural occurrence in adolescence, distinguished by the fact that it disappears on flexion of the spine.

Symptomatic scoliosis may occur because of inequality in the length of the legs, and consequently it disappears when the leg lengths are equalised, or when the patient sits down.

'Sciatic scoliosis' is a term applied to the lateral tilt of the spine which may accompany an acute lumbar intervertebral disc protrusion. It is due to muscle spasm which disappears when the underlying cause has been treated. There are a variety of other less common causes of transient symptomatic scoliosis.

True structural scoliosis is always accompanied by rotation of the vertebrae. There is an extensive and detailed classification, only a few examples of which are shown here.

410

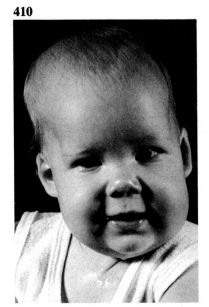

411

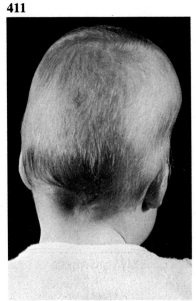

412

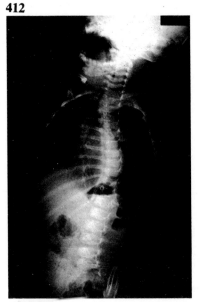

410–412 Infantile idiopathic scoliosis: the curvature is continuous from the top of the head through to the cervical and dorsal regions of the spine. The shape of the head in this condition shows characteristic plagiocephaly.

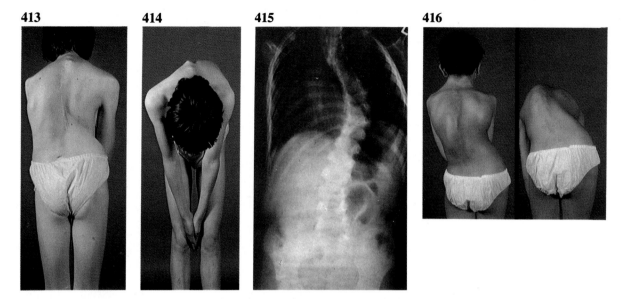

413–416 Idiopathic scoliosis. The commonest variety and usually presents in adolescence. Rotation of the vertebrae and ribcage becomes obvious when the patient flexes the spine. The radiographs show no abnormality apart from the curvature and rotation.

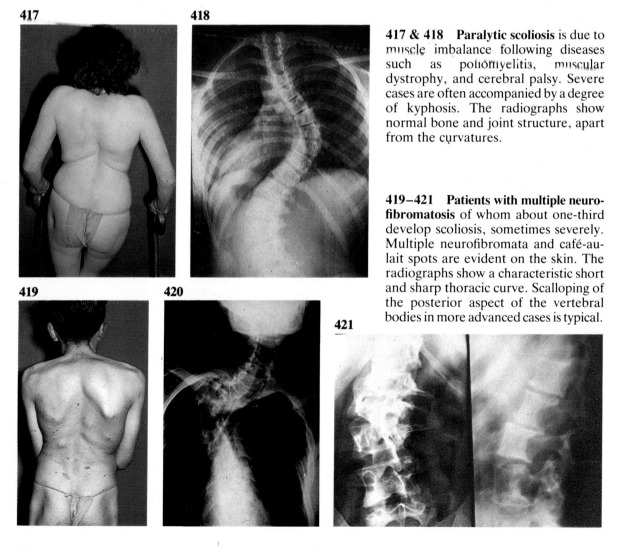

417 & 418 Paralytic scoliosis is due to muscle imbalance following diseases such as poliomyelitis, muscular dystrophy, and cerebral palsy. Severe cases are often accompanied by a degree of kyphosis. The radiographs show normal bone and joint structure, apart from the curvatures.

419–421 Patients with multiple neurofibromatosis of whom about one-third develop scoliosis, sometimes severely. Multiple neurofibromata and café-au-lait spots are evident on the skin. The radiographs show a characteristic short and sharp thoracic curve. Scalloping of the posterior aspect of the vertebral bodies in more advanced cases is typical.

Lumbar intervertebral disc protrusion

Although an intervertebral disc may protrude in any direction and at any level of the spine, by far the commonest site giving rise to symptoms is in the lower lumbar region. The syndrome of 'lumbago-sciatica' develops.

422

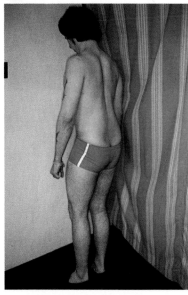

422 Obliteration of normal lumbar lordosis and the patient stands leaning forwards.

423

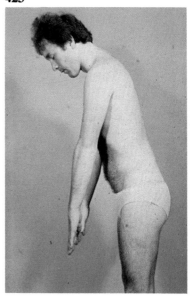

423 Restriction of forward flexion. On attempting to touch his toes the lumbar spine hardly flexes at all and the movement is grossly restricted.

424

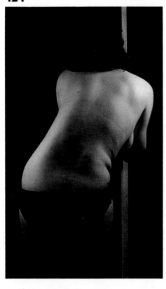

424 'Sciatic scoliosis': when the patient bends forwards there may be a marked tilt of his body, usually away from the affected side. This patient has acute left sciatica. Note the very marked 'list' to the right, and the absence of any vertebral rotation.

425

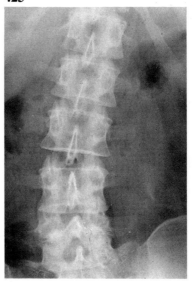

425 Radiograph shows tilting of the spine without vertebral rotation.

426 Straight-leg-raising test (i). The examiner raises the unaffected leg; the range is normal but at the extreme the patient may experience pain in the opposite leg.

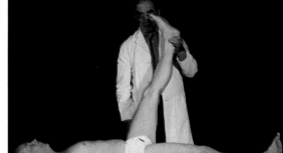

427 Straight-leg-raising test (ii). There is considerable restriction in passive straight leg raising on the affected side due to pain and muscle spasm caused by nerve root tension.

427

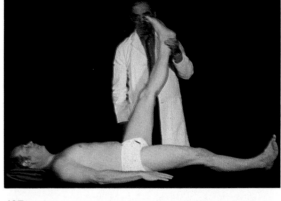

428 Straight-leg-raising test (iii). Lasegue's test: At the position of maximum straight leg raising, the ankle and foot are passively dorsiflexed causing marked increase of pain.

428

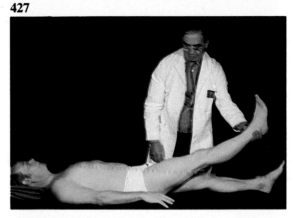

429 Straight-leg-raising test (iv). Naffziger's test: Tension on the nerve root is further increased by passive flexion of neck on trunk.

429

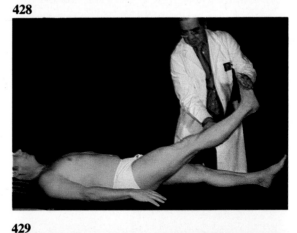

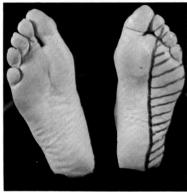

430 The area of altered sensibility corresponds to the nerve root involved. In this patient the S1 nerve root has been compressed by a lumbosacral disc protrusion causing diminished sensibility in the shaded area of the foot.

431

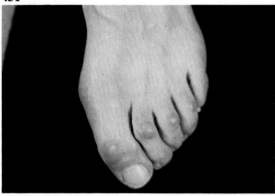

431 Severe disc protrusion eight years previously. Weakness of the intrinsic muscles of the foot (S1) has led to clawing of the toes. Although reflex changes are frequently noted, muscle paralysis is rare.

432

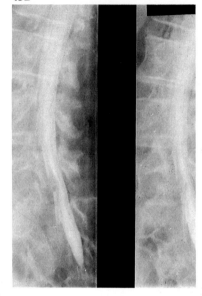

432 Radiculograph to show interruption of the flow of contrast material in the dural sheath of L5 nerve root.

434

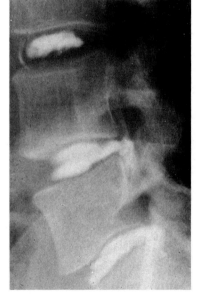

433

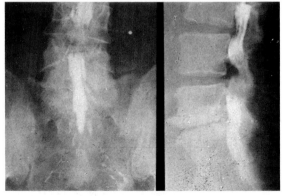

433 A massive disc protrusion L4/5. Although the L5/S1 shows old damage, the cause of this patient's symptoms, confirmed on myelography, is a massive posterior protrusion at L4/5 causing marked interruption of flow of the contrast material.

434 Discography. The nucleus pulposus of an intervertebral disc is under considerable physiological tension. It may protrude through the vertebral endplate or backwards through a ruptured annulus where it is in immediate anatomical relation with one or more spinal nerve roots.

Spondylolisthesis

Spondylolisthesis is a forward shift of a vertebra upon the one below it. It is most common at the lower two lumbar intervertebral joints L4/5, L5/S1. The posterior facet joints – either through single or repeated stresses or by degeneration – fail to provide the normal locking mechanism which prevent the vertebrae from slipping forwards.

435

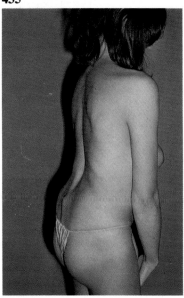

435 Prominent spinous process of S1 and a marked increase of the lumbar lordosis above it.

436

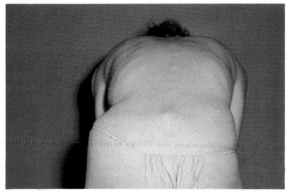

436 On forward flexion the prominent spinous process of S1 is clearly seen. It has – as it were – been left behind by the forward slide of the vertebra above it.

437 In an acute phase the patient is unable to flex the lumbar spine and therefore cannot touch her toes.

437

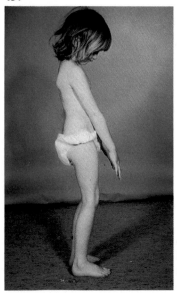

438

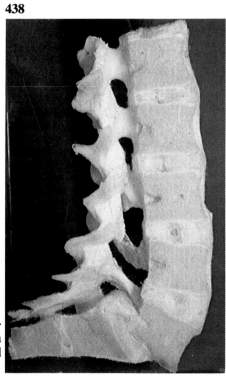

438 Lumbosacral spondylolisthesis. Sagittal sections of a specimen show the pathological anatomy.

439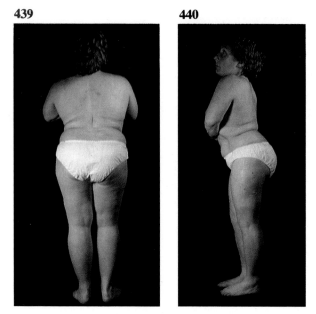

440

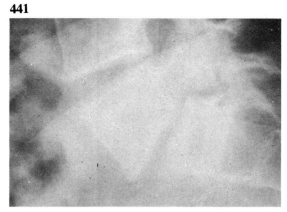

441 Radiographs to show forward slip of L5 on the sacrum in degenerative spondylolisthesis. The posterior facet joints as well as the intervertebral disc are markedly degenerate.

439 **Flank creases** are characteristic.

440 The buttocks protrude backwards, the abdomen protrudes forwards, and the deep flank creases are evident.

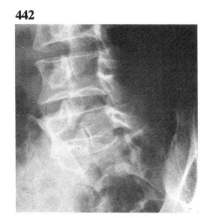

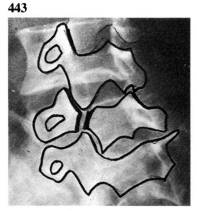

442 **The spondylolitic type of spondylolisthesis** is well demonstrated in oblique radiographs of the lumbar spine. The lamina and posterior facet joints imitate a series of 'scottie dogs'. The third dog from above has apparently been decapitated due to stress fractures.

443 **An outline of the 'dogs':** the interruption of the neck of the central dog almost certainly represents a stress fracture (spondylolysis).

The shoulder region
Acromioclavicular joint

444

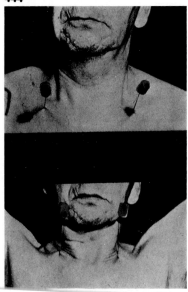

445

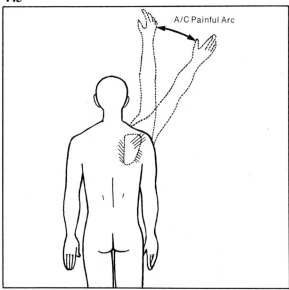

A/C Painful Arc

444 Axial rotation of the clavicle. Two wires have been placed into the inner ends of both clavicles; when the arms are fully abducted the wires are seen to point vertically upwards showing that during abduction the clavicles have rotated almost 90° in the coronal plane.

445 Acromioclavicular painful arc: Because abduction of the arm is accompanied by rotation of the clavicle the pain of acromioclavicular joint disorder is maximal at the extreme of abduction.

446

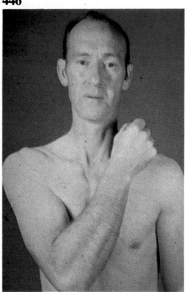

446 Occupational arthritis of the right acromioclavicular joint in a steelworker. The lump seen on top of the right shoulder is an adventitious bursa overlying an osteophyte.

447

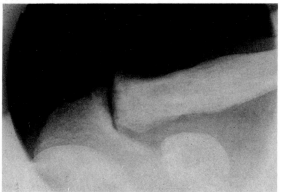

447 Typical degenerative arthritis affecting the right acromioclavicular joint with loss of joint space, sclerosis, pseudocyst formation and superior osteophytes is seen in the radiograph.

448

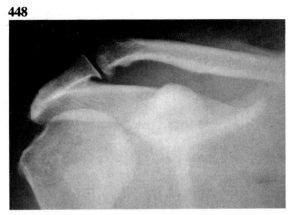

448 Severe acromioclavicular degenerative arthritis.

449

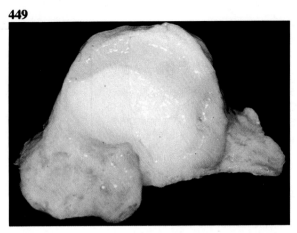

449 The intra-articular meniscus with cyst formation removed from the same patient.

450

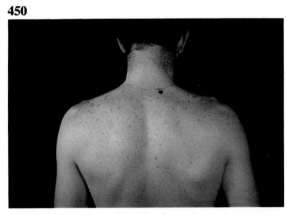

450 & 451 Subluxation of the right acromioclavicular joint due to a trivial injury long since forgotten. The prominent out end of the clavicle is best seen from behind with the arms in full adduction.

451

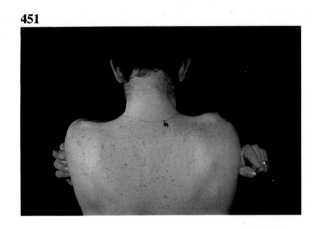

452

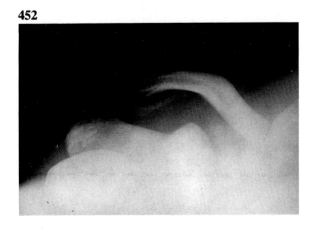

452 Radiograph of the same patient. New bone formation is seen on the undersurface of the clavicle from which the periosteum had been stripped.

Subacromial joint

453 A normal shoulder. The anatomical area bounded above by the acromion and the coraco-acromial ligament, and below by the head and tuberosities of the humerus, has been variously designated. It is most conveniently considered as a surgical joint, called here: The subacromial joint.

454 & 455 The joint space is formed by the sub-acromial bursa whose floor is centrally tethered to the tendons of the rotator muscle cuff. The extent of the bursa which serves as the synovial lining of the subacromial joint.

453

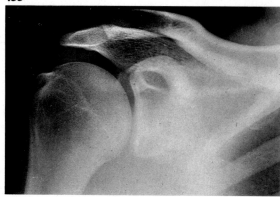

454

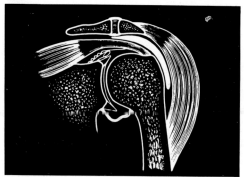

455

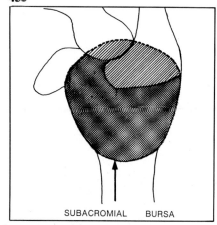

SUBACROMIAL   BURSA

457

456

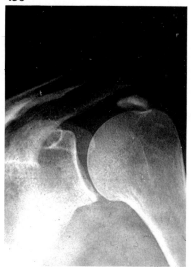

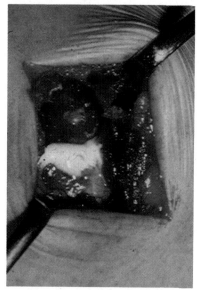

456 Acute calcific bursitis. Radiograph of a patient with intense pain in the shoulder shows a deposition of radio-opaque calcium salts. The deposit consists essentially of calcium apatite with a surrounding inflammatory reaction.

457 The consistency of the calcific deposit at operation is very variable. In the acute phase it is under considerable tension and is virtually a sterile chemical abscess.

458

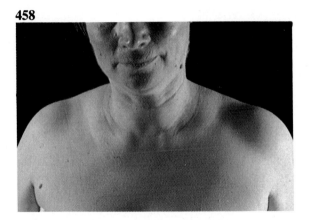

458 Chronic subacromial bursitis. The alteration of contour due to the enlargement of the subacromial bursa on the left in a case of rheumatoid arthritis.

459

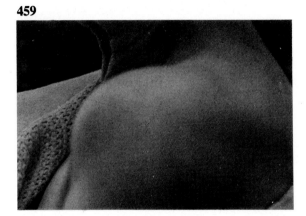

459 Subacromial bursitis highlighted from the side.

460

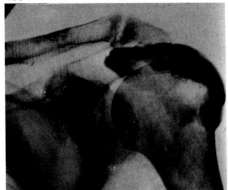

460 Contrast medium injected to produce a subacromial bursograph.

461

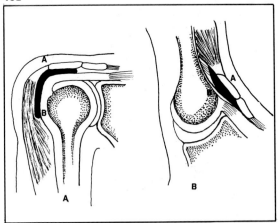

462

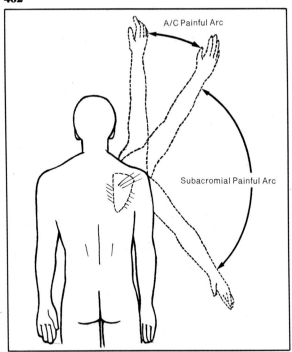

A/C Painful Arc

Subacromial Painful Arc

461 Note how the walls of the subacromial bursa glide with abduction of the shoulder so that points A and B come to lie opposite each other at the extremes of movement. The same gliding takes place during both abduction and rotation.

462 The subacromial painful arc. Gliding of the bursal walls and simultaneous outward rotation of the head of the humerus to achieve abduction starts at about 40° and is complete at about 120°. Any inflammatory disorder of the subacromial joint therefore causes a painful arc of abduction between 40° and 120°. Below and above these points the pain is less pronounced.

463 Before any radiographic changes are evident, soft-tissue impingement can be demonstrated by injecting contrast material. Here the supraspinatus tendon is seen kinked to a right angle by impingement of the coraco-acromial ligament. A line imagined from the tip of the coracoid to the acromion demonstrates the site of impingement.

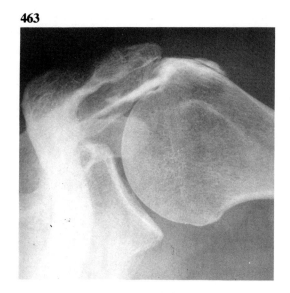

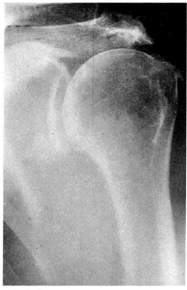

464 Intermediate stage of subacromial arthritis, illustrating that the same changes occur as in other synovial joints. There is sclerosis and osteophyte formation on either side, at the acromion and greater tuberosity.

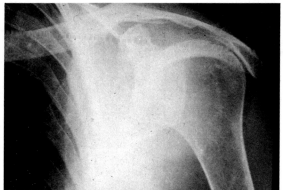

465 Subacromial degenerative arthritis in its final stage in which the intervening soft-tissues give way and the atrophic tuberosity area of the humerus comes to form a secondary articulation with the undersurface of the acromion.

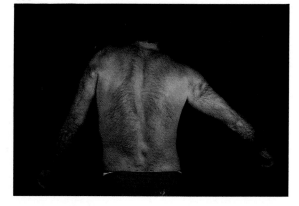

466 Rupture of the rotator cuff. The patient is unable to abduct his arm without hunching the shoulder. There is a reversal of normal scapulo-humeral rhythm. Passive movements are full.

Varieties of rupture of the rotator cuff.

467

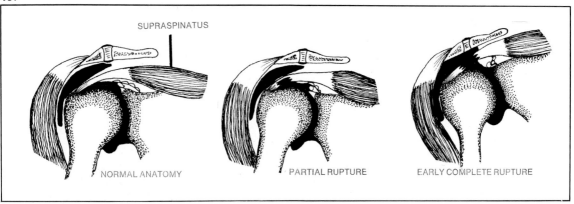

SUPRASPINATUS

NORMAL ANATOMY   PARTIAL RUPTURE   EARLY COMPLETE RUPTURE

468

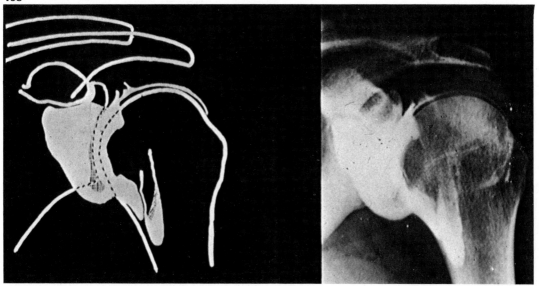

468   Normal arthrograph of the shoulder joint. Contrast material in the glenohumeral joint: it outlines the articular cartilage of the head of the humerus, the subcoracoid bursa, the inferior joint recess, and the tendon sheath of the long head biceps.

469

469   Total rupture of the rotator cuff. In this arthrograph of the shoulder the contrast medium escapes into the subacromial bursa, and outlines both joint and bursa.

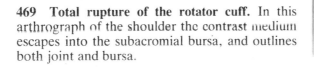

470 **An acute massive rupture of rotator cuff** demonstrated at operation. The cuff has been retracted to show the underlying bare head of the humerus.

470

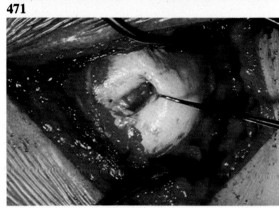

471 **Chronic attrition rupture of the rotator cuff.** Healing has taken place with a tough fibrous ring leaving a small defect between subacromial bursa and shoulder joint. Normal movements have returned but a painful arc of abduction persists.

471

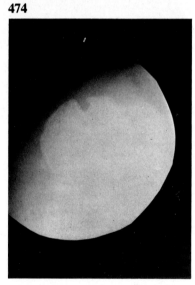

472

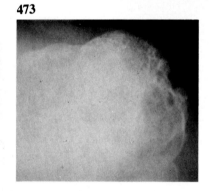

473

473 Radiograph of the patient's shoulder: a tangential view of the sulcus for LHB between the greater and lesser tuberosities of the humerus. Note the marked osteophyte and pseudocyst formation of degenerative joint disease.

474

472 **Rupture of the tendon of the long head of biceps.** This may occur suddenly or imperceptibly without the patient's knowledge.

474 **A normal bicipital sulcus** for comparison.

Glenohumeral joint

475

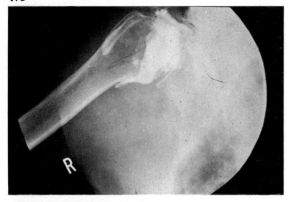

475 'The frozen shoulder'. An acutely painful and increasingly stiff shoulder is designated as a 'frozen shoulder' providing no cause can be found. An arthrograph of a 'frozen shoulder' in which there is one clear abnormality compared to the normal arthrograph, i.e. the joint space is considerably reduced, accepting only about 6–8ml of contrast fluid compared to the 25–30ml of fluid accepted into a normal shoulder joint. Reduction of the joint space is also evidenced by the obliteration of the inferior joint recess.

476

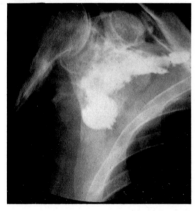

477

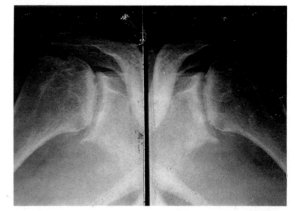

476 Radiograph of the same patient carried out immediately following manipulation of the shoulder to demonstrate how the joint capsule has been ruptured and the contrast medium flows out freely into the soft tissues in the subscapular region.

477 Rheumatoid arthritis. The glenohumeral joint is only rarely affected by any form of arthritis. Rheumatoid disease is by far the commonest cause.

478

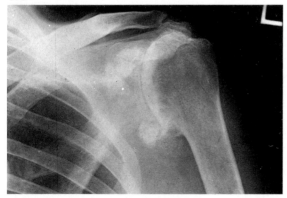

479

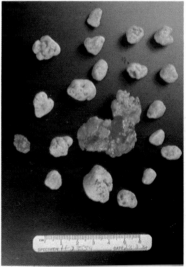

478 Synovial osteochondromatosis of the glenohumeral joint.

479 Multiple osteochondromata removed at operation.

480

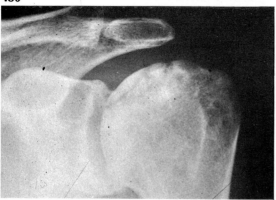

481

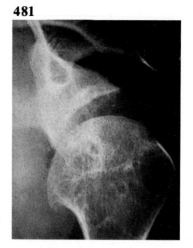

480 Caisson disease (dysbaric osteonecrosis). The shoulder of a tunnel worker. This occupational disease is uncommon. When it does occur, however, the shoulders are frequently affected. A lozenge shaped infarct is seen on the superomedial aspect of the head of the humerus which is due to avascular necrosis from gas embolism.

481 Haemophilic arthropathy. Shoulder of a patient suffering from another rare cause of gleno-humeral arthritis.

482

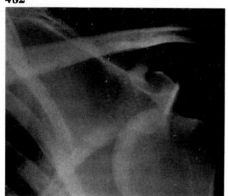

Shoulder instability

482 Recurrent anterior dislocation of the shoulder joint is a common disorder. The basic pathology consists of a detachment of the capsule from the front of the shoulder joint at the time of the original dislocation, usually combined with an impaction fracture in the posterior part of the head of the humerus.

483

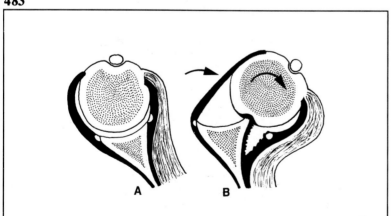

484

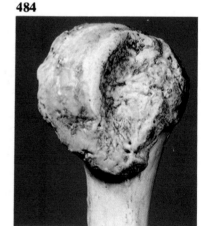

483 To show how the head of the humerus is rotated out and causes a detachment of the capsule, labrum glenoidale and periosteum from the neck of the scapula.

484 Hills-Sachs lesion probably better termed as the Broca lesion, since he was the first to describe it. Specimen of an old recurrent disloca-tion of the shoulder showing the impaction fracture of the posterior part of the head of the humerus.

485

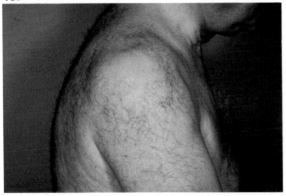

485 Posterior dislocation of the shoulder joint. The clinical appearances are very deceptive. Careful inspection reveals a bulge at the back of the shoulder, which is the head of the humerus.

486

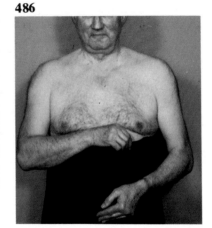

486 Fixed internal rotation of the shoulder is the single most important diagnostic sign.

487

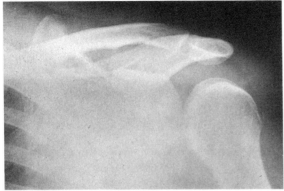

487 The standard anteroposterior radiograph can be very deceiving.

488

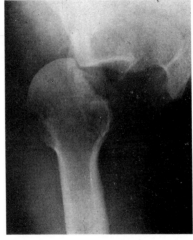

488 A lateral radiograph of the same shoulder to reveal the posterior dislocation.

489

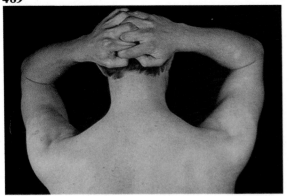

490

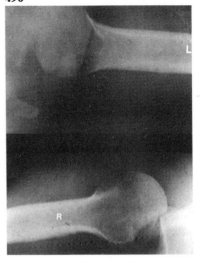

489 & 490 Habitual, bilateral, posterior dislocation of shoulders.

491 Neuralgic amyotrophy (Paralytic brachial neuritus or shoulder girdle paralysis). A presumed virus disease of acute onset leading to variable peripheral nerve damage. This patient has a wasted and completely paralysed deltoid muscle (see **176**).

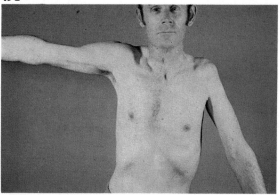

492 Deltoid paralysis following fracture dislocation of the right shoulder joint. The hollow seen on the outer aspect of the shoulder is due to downward subluxation of the head of the humerus.

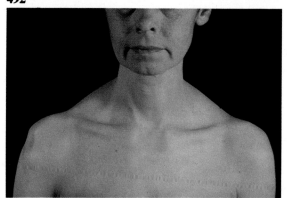

493 Facio-scapular muscular dystrophy (see also **184–6**). The muscles controlling the scapula have become gradually paralysed. On the left side the condition is untreated and the original clinical signs remain: wasting of shoulder girdle musculature, winging of the scapula, loss of range and power of abduction of the shoulder. Compare the right side on which an operation has been performed to fuse the scapula to the chest wall: improved stability of the scapula and movements of the right shoulder have been achieved.

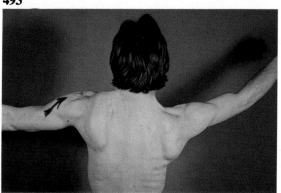

494 Contracture of deltoid due to intramuscular injections. This patient was given a series of intramuscular injections of antibiotics as a result of which some of the muscle was destroyed and replaced by fibrous tissue. On attempting to bring her arms to her side the shortened and tethered deltoid muscles do not allow normal adduction at the glenohumeral joints and the scapulae are forced to rotate early. The scapulae become prominent and simulate the winging of serratus anterior paralysis.

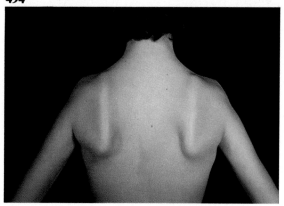

The elbow region

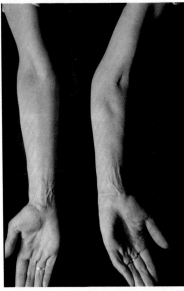

495 Cubitus valgus. This deformity is due to injury causing an immediate deformity by malunion of a fracture, or a gradually developing deformity due to damage and premature arrest of the lower humeral growth plate. It is the classical (but not the commonest) cause of tardy ulnar palsy (*vi*), because the ulnar nerve now has to take a longer course behind the medial epicondyle.

496

497

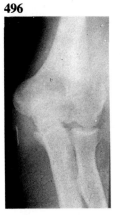
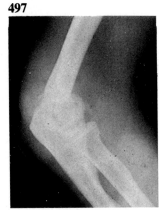

496 & 497 Cubitus valgus due to a malunited fracture of the lateral condyle of the humerus.

498

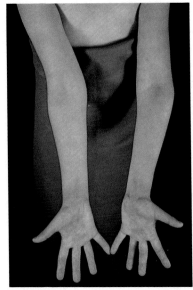

498 Cubitus varus. This causes little functional impairment but relief is often sought on aesthetic grounds.

499

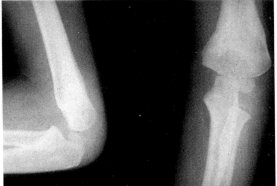

499 Radiograph shows cubitus varus due to a malunited supracondylar fracture.

115

500 & 501   Supracondylar spur. This is a rare but interesting cause of neurovascular compression in the arm causing symptoms which simulate the carpal tunnel syndrome. The supracondylar process is an anatomical atavism.

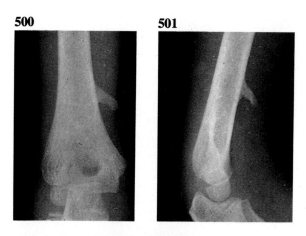

502   Brachial arteriograph showing high division of the brachial artery with impaired filling of the ulnar branch due to compression.

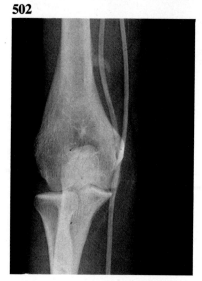

503   The area displayed at operation: from the tip of the spur the ligament of Struthers can be seen to run downwards towards the left crossing over the median nerve and ulnar vessels.

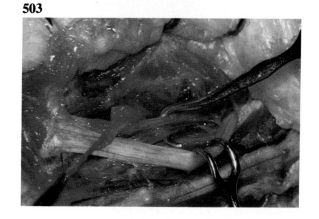

Tardy ulnar palsy 504–512.

504 The ulnar nerve is pushed medially and backwards against the arch of a fibrous tunnel straddling the two heads of origin of flexor carpi ulnaris. At the site of constriction there is an indentation of the nerve and immediately proximal to it a swelling: the neuroma. The swelling is more accurately described, however, as a glioma due to intraneural fibrosis.

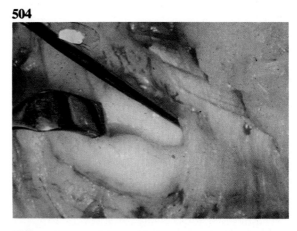

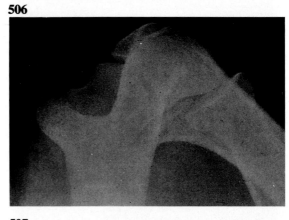

505 The ulnar tunnel has been divided and the nerve now lies free. The ischaemic area of the nerve compressed can clearly be seen.

506 Tangential radiograph to show the normal ulnar groove behind the medial condyle of the humerus.

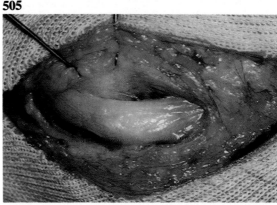

507 Radiograph of a patient suffering from tardy ulnar palsy due to encroachment on the ulnar groove by osteophytes.

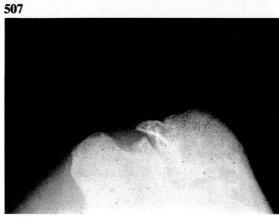

508

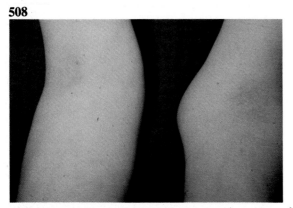

509

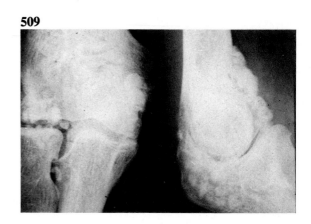

508 & 509 Synovial chondromatosis. Pronounced soft tissue swelling over the medial aspect of the left elbow. Radiographs reveal the multiple chondromata.

510

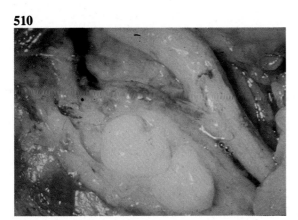

510 The chondromata escaped when the synovial membrane adjacent to the ulnar nerve was incised.

511

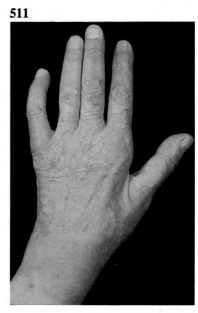

511 Intrinsic muscle wasting of the hand in a case of tardy ulnar palsy.

512

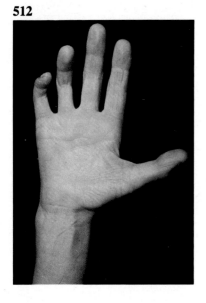

512 Ulnar claw hand due to advanced ulnar palsy by compression of the ulnar nerve at the elbow. Paradoxically, the deformity of the hand is greater when the lesion is more distal. Claw hand due to a low ulnar lesion is depicted in **584**.

513

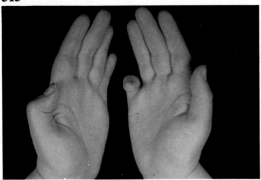

513 Congenital contracture of the little finger.
Distinguished from other finger contractures by its presence from birth, and the fact that it is always the proximal IP joint of the little finger which is alone affected.

514

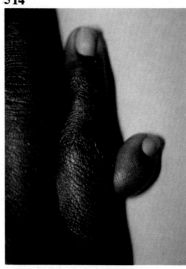

514 Supernumerary digit.

515

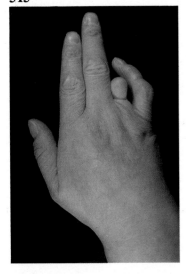

516

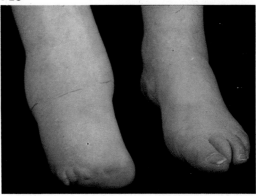

515 & 516 Congenital amputation of the fingers and toes. Its occurrence in both hand and foot of the same patient show it to be a developmental disorder rather than due to intrauterine damage.

517

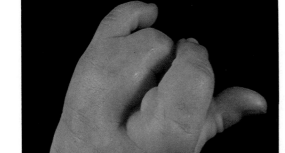

517 Congenital lobster claw deformity.

518

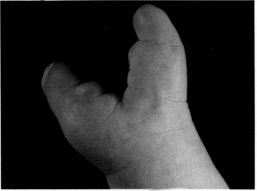

518 There is often very good movement of the 'claw' with good function.

519

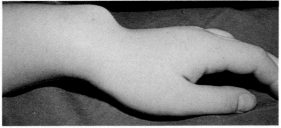

520

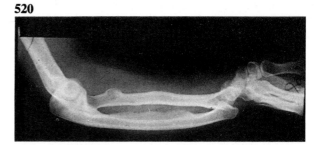

519 Madelung's deformity of the wrist. This usually becomes manifest at about ten years-of-age and increases until growth is completed. It may be congenital but is often due to injury affecting the lower radius growth plate.

520 Radiograph of the forearm to show the relatively long ulna in Madelung's deformity.

521

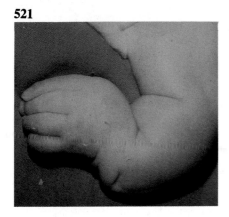

522

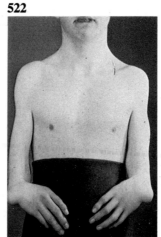

523

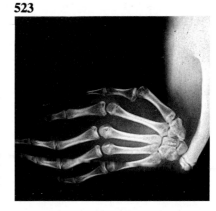

523 Radial clubhand in which, uncommonly, the thumb element remains.

521 Radial clubhand. The whole of the pre-axial (radial) side of the forearm is underdeveloped or absent. The thumb is usually absent.

522 Bilateral radial clubhand showing the considerable underdevelopment of the forearm between elbow and hand.

524

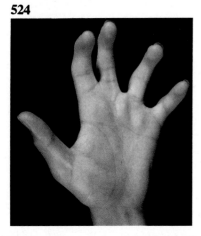

525

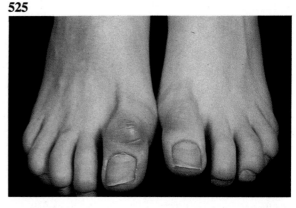

524 & 525 Arachnodaktyly ('spider fingers'). The long and tapering fingers may indicate general systemic abnormalities associated with this condition.

The feet of the same patient. Arachnodaktyly is probably in the same family as Marfan's syndrome, a disorder of autosomal dominant inheritance. Dislocation of the lens of the eye, aortic aneurysm and scoliosis are some of the associated abnormalities.

526

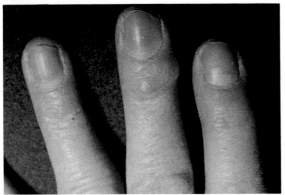

527

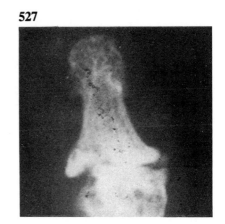

526 & 527   Cysts on the dorsum of the terminal finger joint are due to synovial hypertrophy and protrusion from the diseased joints. This is more common in generalised osteoarthritis than in rheumatoid arthritis.

528–531   Rheumatoid arthritis of the wrist and fingers. These joints are often the first clinically affected in rheumatoid disease. The metacarpophalangeal joints are commonly affected. Destructive arthropathy is seen in the radiographs. A profile view of the hands shows the flexor tendons of the little fingers of the hands have suffered spontaneous rupture.

528

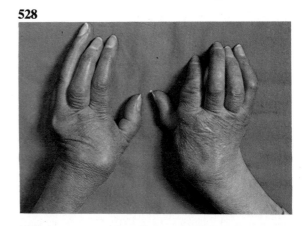

529

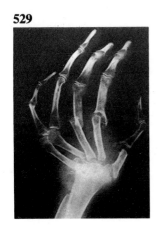

530

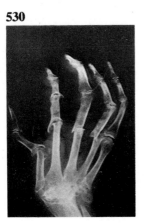

531

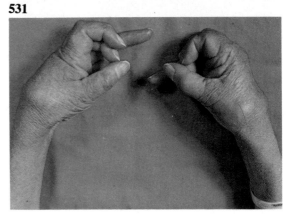

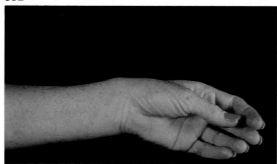

532

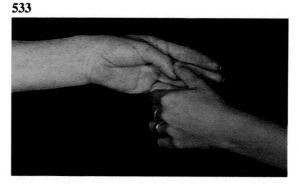

533

532 De Quervain's disease. Stenosing teno-synovitis commonly occurs in the extensor retina-culum tunnel through which the long thumb tendons run. The swelling is seen in profile on the radial aspect of the wrist.

533 Passive ulnar adduction of the thumb sharply aggravates the pain.

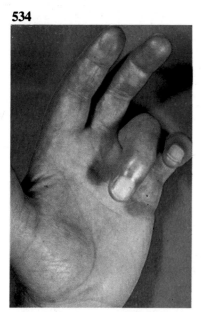

534

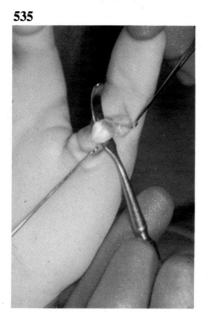

535

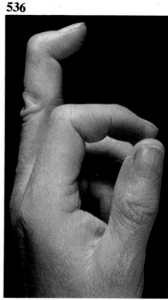

536

534 Trigger finger: stenosing tendosynovitis at the entrance to the fibrous flexor sheath causes a fibrous nodule to develop in the long flexor tendons. The swelling snaps to and fro through the entrance of the sheath, causing the finger to trigger. It may be either an early manifestation of rheumatoid disease or it may be occupational in origin.

535 Trigger thumb: flexor pollicis longus tendon is displayed at the entrance to the fibrous flexor sheath. It occurs either in the newborn: owing to the foetal position of the thumb clasped into the hand; or as an early mani-festation of rheumatoid disease; or from occupational causes.

536 Mallet finger: rupture of the insertion of the terminal extensor tendon slip sometimes with a tiny fragment of bone. It may occur from trivial injury.

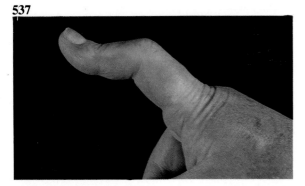

537 **Boutonnière deformity:** rupture of the central slip of the extensor tendon over the proximal IP joint, allowing the head of the proximal phalanx to buttonhole through the dorsum. The lateral slips of the extensor tendon mechanism are displaced to the sides and maintain the deformity.

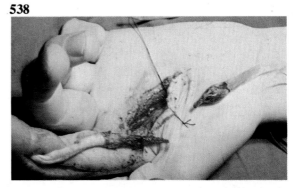

538 **Ruptured flexor digitorum profundus** to the index finger. Rupture of flexor tendons occur at the wrist in rheumatoid arthritis although it is less common than rupture of extensor tendons. Vascularisation of the diseased tendon preceding rupture can clearly be seen.

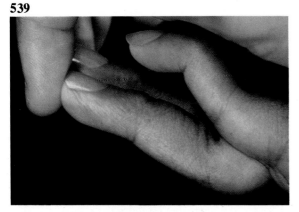

539 **Swan-neck deformity:** disruption of the volar plate of the proximal IP joint, sometimes with rupture of the insertion of flexor sublimis.

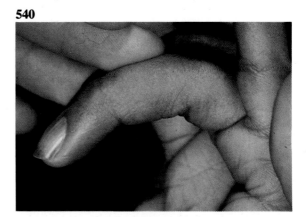

540 The deformity is immediately correctable by passive flexion of the proximal IP joint.

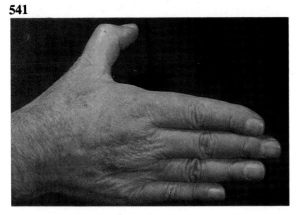

541 **Ruptured extensor pollicis longus tendon.**

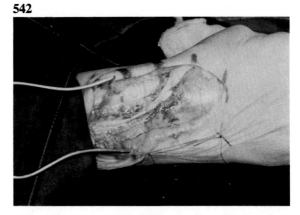

542 The ruptured EPL tendon displayed at operation. It may occur either spontaneously in rheumatoid arthritis, or after a Colles' fracture due to attrition over a bony fragment on the dorsum of the radius.

543

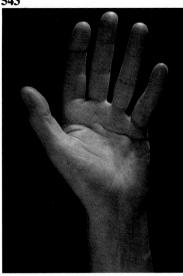

543 & 544 Dupuytren's contracture. Thickening and contracture of the palmar fascia which involves skin, and running across the proximal joints of the fingers causes fixed contracture. In early Dupuytren's contracture only one finger, often the little finger, is initially affected. It is ten times more common in men and is probably of sex-linked autosomal dominant inheritance. There may be progressive contracture of all the fingers.

544

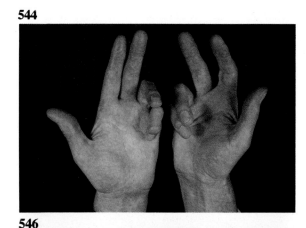

545

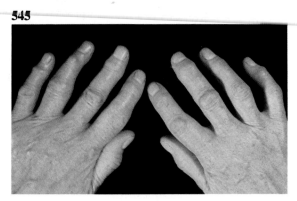

545 Garrod's Pads. Thickening of the subcutaneous tissues on the dorsum of the proximal IP joints seen in association with Dupuytren's contracture. This patient also had Heberden's nodes over the terminal phalanges of the fingers: an indication of primary generalised osteoarthritis.

546

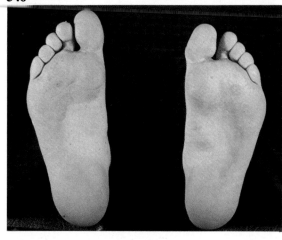

546 Dupuytren's contracture. Fibrous nodular thickening is sometimes seen in the plantar fascia.

547

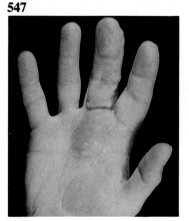

548

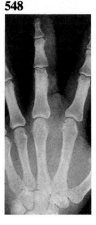

547 & 548 Lipofibromatosis of the hand. A rare and locally invasive tumour simulating Dupuytren's contracture. Nodular soft tissue shadows at the base of the middle finger are revealed in the radiographs.

Volkmann's ischaemic contracture

549 & 550 When the wrist is extended the fingers are strongly forced into flexion by the shortened flexor muscles; when the wrist is flexed the fingers can be straightened.

549

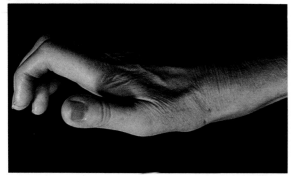

550

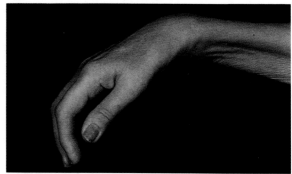

551 Ischaemia of the forearm muscles and nerves. The fingers are flexed and there is marked wasting of the intrinsic muscles of the hand.

552 The forearm muscles seen at operation. A segment of the muscle bulk has been replaced by scar tissue.

551

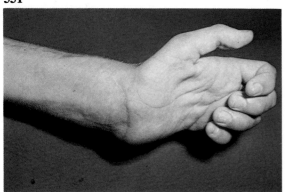

552

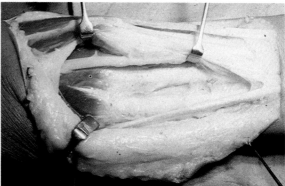

553

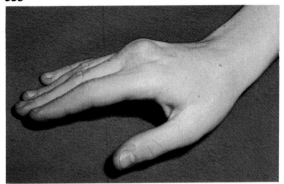

554

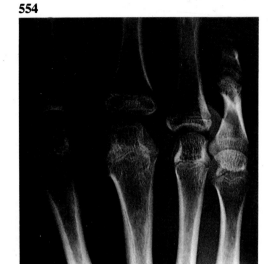

553 & 554 Enchondroma of the hand. Isolated enlargement of the neck of the middle metacarpal bone. Expansion of the neck and shaft of the metacarpal due to a simple cartilage tumour.

555

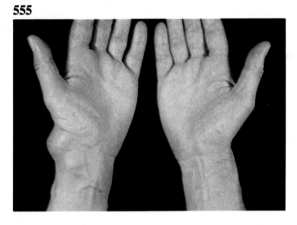

556

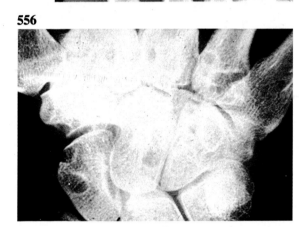

555 & 556 Pigmented villonodular synovitis of the wrist. The wrist is generally swollen and a number of globular tumours are seen on the radial aspect.

The tissue is solid but soft in consistency. Radiography shows that PVNS may cause multiple lytic erosions in the bones related to the affected synovial membrane.

557

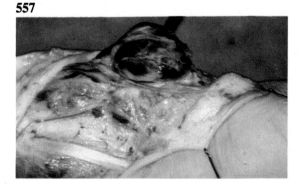

557 At operation the process is seen to involve not only the synovial membrane of the wrist, but also of the nearby extensor tendon sheaths.

558

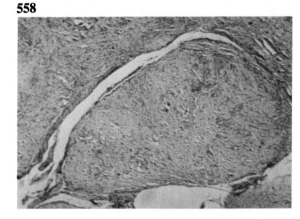

558 PVNS removed at operation. The blue-stained areas contain iron pigment. *(× 100)*

559

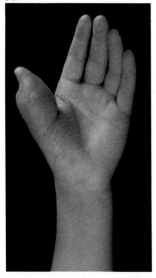

560

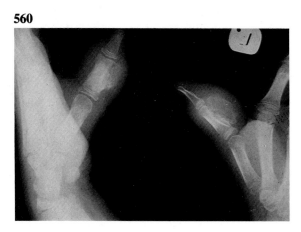

559 & 560   Implantation dermoid cyst. A solid soft tissue mass enlarging almost the whole of the left thumb. There were no signs of active inflammation, and no history of trauma was recalled. A calcified mass which appears to have eroded the proximal phalanx can be seen in the radiograph. The diagnosis of an implantation dermoid cyst was confirmed after excision of the mass.

561

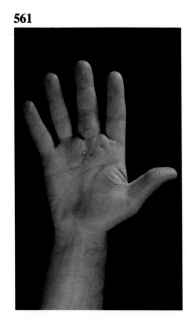

562

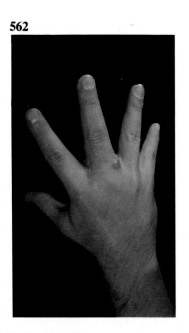

563

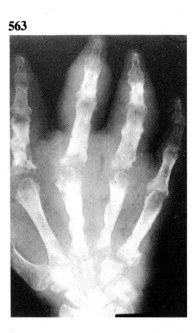

561–563   Madura hand: fungus infection by the mycetoma organism is commoner in the foot but is occasionally seen in the hand. The hand shows the typical subcutaneous nodules at the base of the middle finger. The radiograph shows an advanced case of Madura hand.

564 Raynaud's phenomenon. Intermittent spasm of the small peripheral arterioles initiated by cold, causing blanching of fingers and toes. It may be due to a variety of causes. In severe cases, trophic changes and even gangrene may supervene. One cause is the prolonged use of vibrating tools.

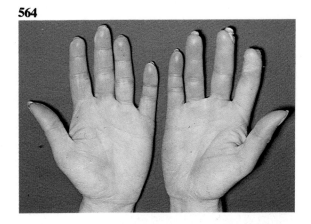

564

565 Soft tissue calcification and atrophy of terminal digits are seen both in cryopathy and chronic Raynaud's phenomenon.

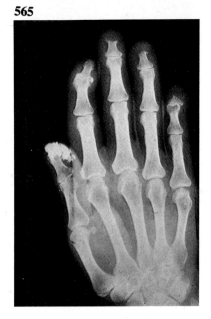

565

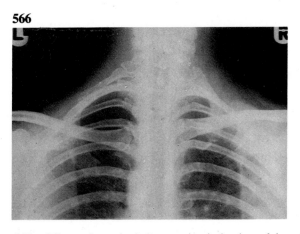

566

566 Bilateral cervical ribs causing irritation of the cervical sympathetic fibres was established as the cause in the radiograph.

Peripheral nerve injury affecting the hand

567

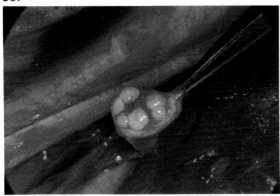

567 Normal nerve bundles in cross-section.

568

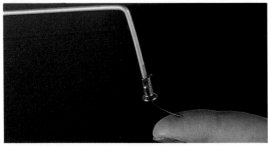

568 Sensory testing of the skin is of critical importance in nerve injuries of the hand. A simple device consists of a piece of O-calibre nylon fixed into a bicycle spoke which has been curved to a right-angle. A pressure equivalent to 1g von Frey hair deforms the nylon.

569 Quinizarine powder turns deep blue when it is moistened by sweat. The area which remains unchanged has therefore been deprived of its normal pseudomotor nerve fibres which are carried in the sensory nerves to their destination. The test outlines the insensitive area of skin in a complete median nerve lesion.

569

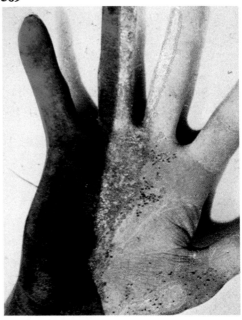

572 Horner's syndrome. The cervical sympathetic fibres traverse T1 nerve root and may be damaged in lower arm palsy, causing ptosis of the eyelid, a constricted pupil, and enophthalmos.

572

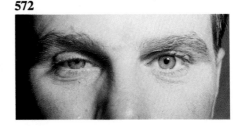

570

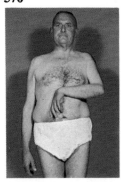

571

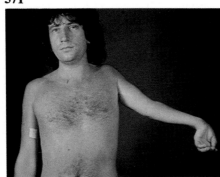

570 Birth injury: upper arm type (Erb's palsy). The arm is held to the side with the forearm in full pronation due to paralysis of the shoulder abductors and forearm supinator muscles supplied by the upper trunk of the brachial plexus C5/6/(7). The unaffected stronger muscles produce the deformity. The typical 'waiter's tip' position.

571 Birth injury: lower arm type (Klumpke). This less common birth injury of the brachial plexus (C8/T1) usually results from a breach delivery with the arm forced above the head. Abduction of the shoulder is possible and the forearm is held in full supination with clawing of the fingers.

573

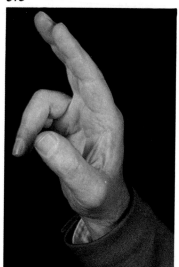

574

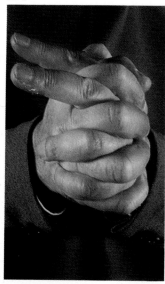

Median nerve injury

A high median nerve lesion causes loss of flexion of the proximal and distal interphalangeal joints of index and middle fingers. In high median nerve paralysis, both long flexors of index and middle fingers fail to flex at the interphalangeal joints on grasping.

573   The hand of benediction.

574   Ochsner's clasping test.

575

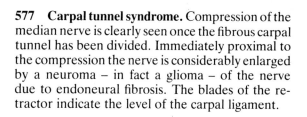

576

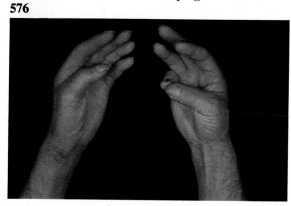

575   Selective wasting of the thenar muscles: the photograph has been specially lighted to show the loss of muscle bulk of abductor pollicis brevis. This may be a valuable sign of median nerve damage, e.g. due to compression at the carpal tunnel.

576   Opposition of the thumb: an early and reliable sign of median nerve damage. Note that the right thumb opposes fully to the little finger, whereas on the left side it fails to do so and less of the thumb nail is visible due to impaired rotation.

577

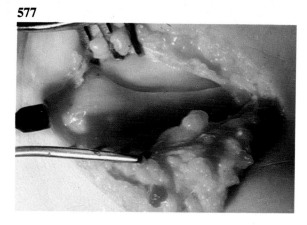

577   Carpal tunnel syndrome. Compression of the median nerve is clearly seen once the fibrous carpal tunnel has been divided. Immediately proximal to the compression the nerve is considerably enlarged by a neuroma – in fact a glioma – of the nerve due to endoneural fibrosis. The blades of the retractor indicate the level of the carpal ligament.

Ulnar nerve injury

578

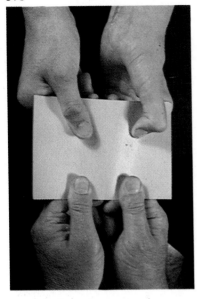

579

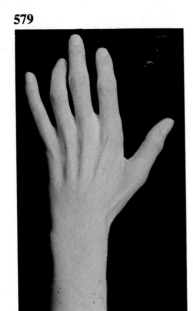

580

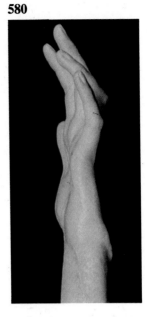

578 Froment's sign: on attempting to grasp the paper between thumb and index finger, the patient's left thumb collapses at the IP joint due to weakness of flexor pollicis brevis.

579 & 580 Wasting of the interossei muscles can be seen by the guttering between the extensor tendons; from the side the attitude of the fingers and the marked wasting of the hypothenar muscles is evident.

581

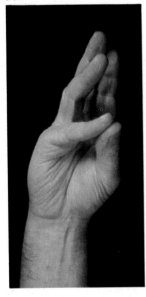

582

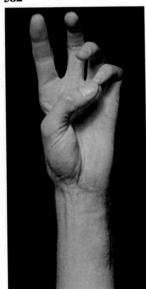

581 Normal opposition of little finger to thumb. Note how flexion takes place at the MP joint and extension at the IP joints.

582 Ulnar paralysis showing abnormal and imperfect opposition of little finger to thumb.

583

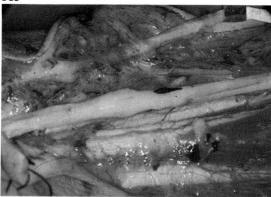

583 'Neuroma'. A lesion in continuity of the ulnar nerve immediately above the wrist. The nerve has been crushed but the perineurium remains intact. At the site of injury the nerve is thinned, but immediately proximal to the injury, it is enlarged by a traumatic 'neuroma'.

585

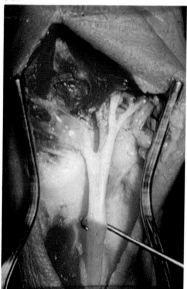

585 Ganglion pressing selectively on the deep branch of the ulnar nerve, as it divided on entering the palm.

584

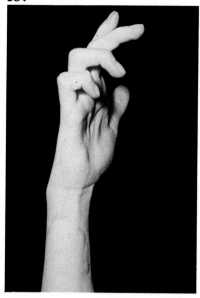

584 A claw-hand following a low ulnar nerve lesion. Note the hyperextension of the MP joints and the marked flexion at the IP joints due to the paralysis of intrinsic muscles and the consequent unopposed action of the long extensor and flexor muscles. The middle and index fingers are less affected because their lumbrical muscles are supplied by the median nerve. Muscle imbalance is therefore less marked in these two fingers.

586

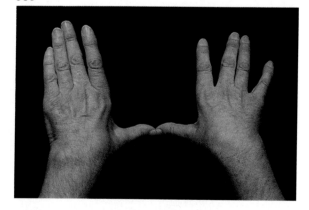

586 Selective wasting of the first dorsal interosseous muscle of the left hand.

587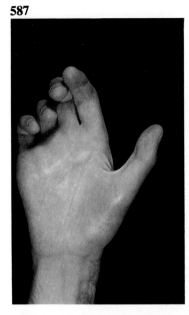

588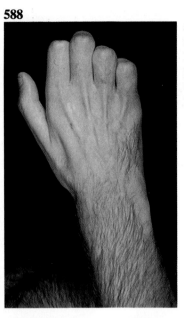

587 & 588 Combined low median and ulnar nerve injury produces the worst form of clawhand. The fixed clawed position of the fingers with thin and atrophic skin is evident. There is severe wasting of all the intrinsic musculature.

589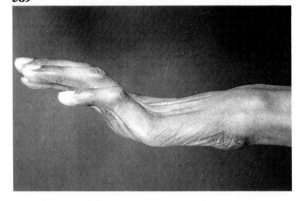

589 Intrinsic muscle paralysis following poliomyelitis in infancy. Hyperextension at the MP and flexion at the proximal IP joints is due to the unopposed action of the long extensor and flexor muscles.

590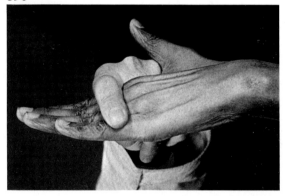

590 The fingers can extend fully when the paralysed intrinsic muscles are passively simulated by the examiner's hand.

591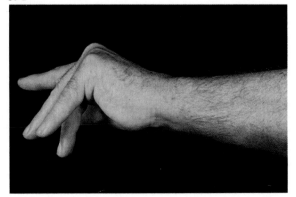

591 Hysterical contraction of the hand. An analysis of the balancing forces of muscle to produce this attitude shows that it is anatomically impossible to explain by any form of nerve damage. It bears some resemblance to Trousseau's sign (main d'accoucher). The condition was, however, unilateral and there was no suggestion of tetany. It is an example of motor hysteria.

The hip joint

592 Hugh Owen-Thomas demonstrating his test to display hidden fixed flexion deformity.

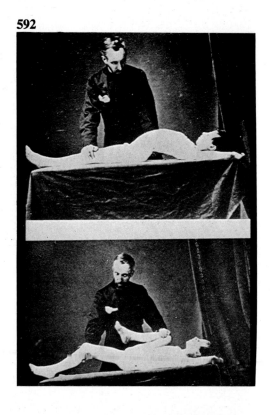

593 & 594 Thomas' test. The patient lies flat on the couch, any fixed flexion deformity is hidden by pelvic tilt increasing the normal lumbar lordosis. When the opposite hip is flexed to obliterate the lumbar lordosis (note the examiner's hand under the lumbar spine to check this) any hidden flexion deformity of the hip becomes apparent.

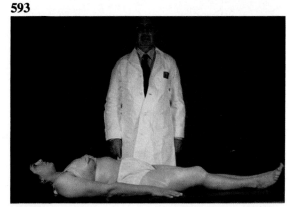

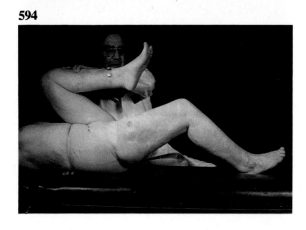

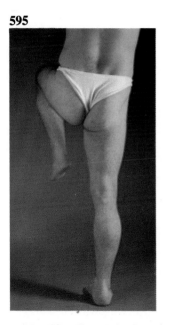

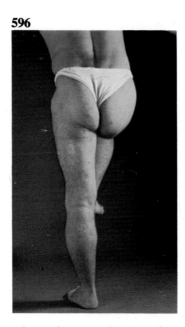

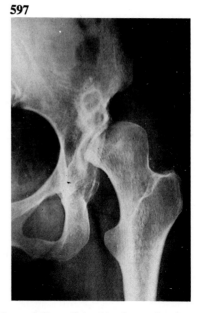

595–597   Trendelenburg's test. When the patient stands on one leg, the stability of the hip depends upon two principal factors: effective muscles between pelvis and greater trochanter, and a stable, centrally placed femoral head. When this mechanism fails for any reason, the test is positive.

The patient stands on the normal leg: his trunk inclines towards the same side, and the pelvis tilts and is stabilised towards the same side causing the other buttock to rise.

Note the position of the gluteal folds. The right hip is stable: the test is negative.

The patient then stands upon the affected side. The stabilising mechanism has failed and the buttock on the opposite side droops downwards; the left hip is unstable: the test is positive.

The cause of failure in this case is due to subluxation of the hip joint so that the fulcrum for the action of the pelvifemoral muscle is lost.

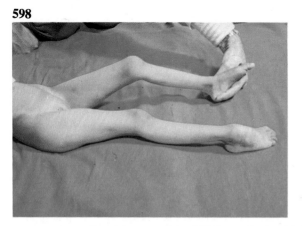

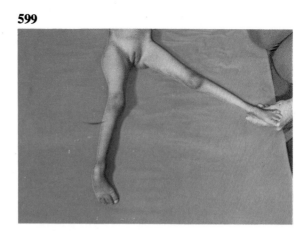

598 & 599   Yount's test. This child has a flexion deformity of both the left hip and knee due to a contracted tensor fascia lata muscle straddling across the hip and knee joints. By abducting the hip to relax tensor fascia lata, the apparent flexion deformity of both the hip and knee diminishes.

Leg length inequality

Inequality of the length of the legs may be due to a wide variety of causes. In its simplest form, it is due to shortening in any part of one leg, or lengthening in any part of the other.

600

601

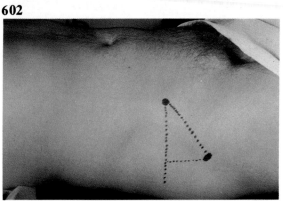

600 & 601 True shortening. When the patient stands erect, the pelvis is tilted due to shortening of the left leg. A block of 5cm underneath the left leg squares the pelvis, indicating true difference in the length of the legs.

602

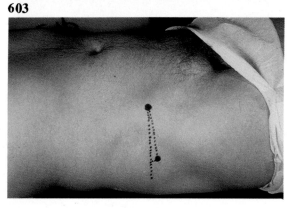

602 Bryant's triangle. Shortening may occur either above or below the greater trochanter, i.e. in the femoral neck and hip joint, or below it. The relation between the anterior superior iliac spine and the tip of the greater trochanter is assessed, by lines drawn from the anterior superior spine vertically downwards and to the tip of the greater trochanter. The base of the triangle is a guide to the neck-shaft angle of the femur. Normally it is more or less an isosceles triangle. In practice, Bryant's triangle does not require to be marked out, but is readily assessed by palpation with the thumb on the anterior superior iliac spine and fingertips on the top of the greater trochanter, the two sides being simultaneously compared.

603

604

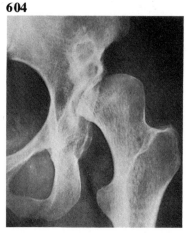

603 & 604 True shortening. The fact that the shortening is sited above the trochanter level is evidenced by the fact that the base of the triangle has been diminished and the trochanter now lies almost vertically below the iliac spine.

604 Radiograph shows the shortening due to upward displacement of the femoral head.

605 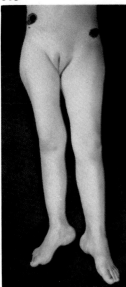   **606**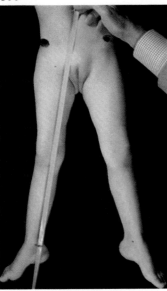

605 & 606   Apparent lengthening. Leg length inequality may be apparent only; fixed adduction deformity at the hip causes apparent shortening, whereas fixed abduction causes apparent lengthening. This child has a fixed abduction deformity of the left hip caused by muscle contracture following poliomyelitis. There is apparent lengthening of the left leg. When the right leg is measured in the same degree of abduction as the left, the leg lengths are seen to be equal.

607 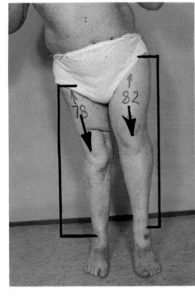   **608**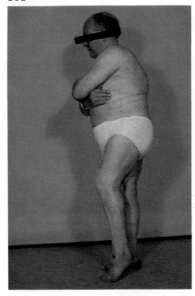

607 & 608   Complex leg inequality. The cause of leg length inequality may be complex; true shortening of one leg may be masked or exceeded by apparent shortening due to fixed deformity of the other hip. This patient stands on the tip of the left toe, suggesting shortening of the left lower limb. The right leg is in fact the shorter. A severe adduction deformity of the left hip more than compensates for the difference.

609

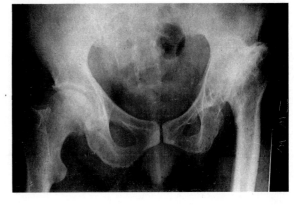

609   Radiographs of the hip to show severe adduction deformity of the left. This caused an apparent shortening of the left leg whereas it was in fact the longer of the two.

610

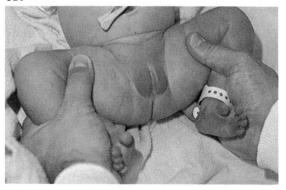

611

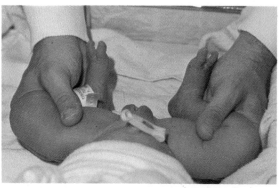

610   Congenital dislocation of the hip. The Barlow test. Newborn infants should be examined for congenital dislocation by one of a number of tests. A positive Barlow test is produced by attempting to relocate the dislocated head by abduction and external rotation.

611   The Ortolani test. The examiner is attempting to relocate a suspected posterior dislocation by forward pressure with the fingers from behind, the thumbs maintaining the hips in abduction. If the sign is positive there is a clunk of re-entry of the head of the femur into the acetabulum on full abduction.

612

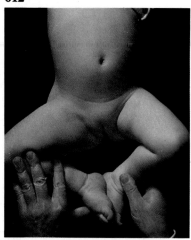

612 & 613   Congenital dislocation of the left hip in a somewhat older infant. There is obvious loss of full abduction in flexion. An unsuccessful attempt to relocate the hip by the Ortolani manoeuvre.

613

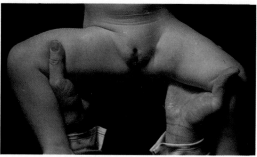

614

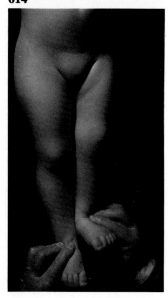

614 & 615   Congenital dislocation of the hip in an older child, illustrating telescoping: the left leg is shortened when the hip is pushed upwards and backwards. This test is probably better done with the hips in the flexed position.

615

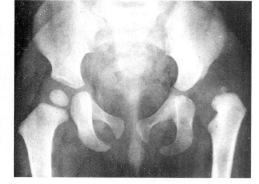

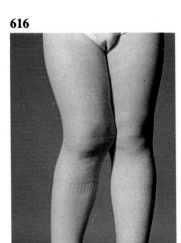

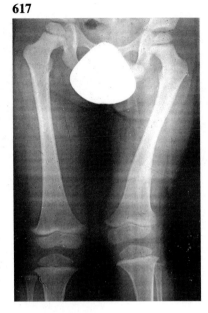

616 & 617 Congenital short femur. The affected leg is on the left. The child prefers to flex his right knee for comfort when standing, because it is relatively too long. The condition varies considerably from almost complete absence of the femur, to relatively slight shortening and alteration of bone texture, as shown on this radiograph.

618

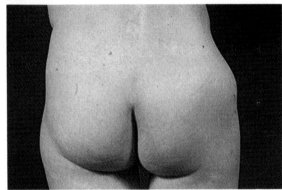

618–620 Congenital coxa vara. This is possibly part of the same spectrum of disorders classified as congenital proximal femoral deficiency.

620

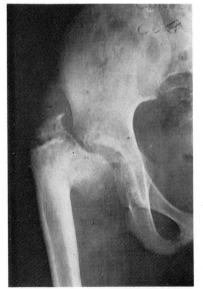

619

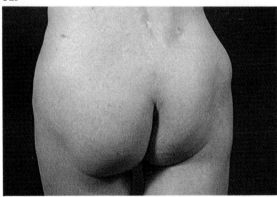

618 & 619 The Trendelenburg test demonstrates positive instability of the right hip. She now takes weight on the abnormal right leg, causing the buttock on the opposite side to droop.

620 Owing to the raised position of the greater trochanter, the pelvifemoral muscles are relatively ineffective and fail to stabilise the hip. This accounts for the positive Trendelenburg test.

621

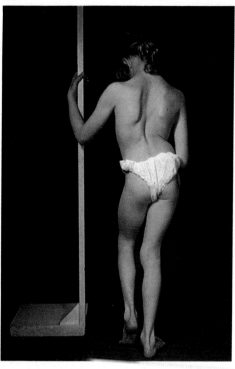

621 Perthes' disease (coxa plana) of the hip is commoner in boys of about five years-of-age. It is transient and self limiting, but alteration of the final shape of the femoral head may lead to hip joint degeneration in later life.

622

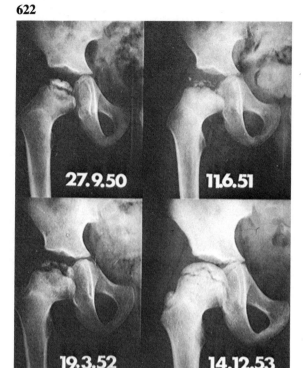

27.9.50   11.6.51

19.3.52   14.12.53

622 Creeping substitution of avascular bone over a three year period from.

623

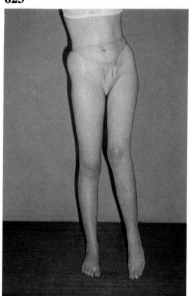

623 & 624 Adolescent coxa vara (slipped epiphysis). The affected left leg is short, externally rotated and adducted. Impairment of normal maturation of the upper femoral epiphysis allows the femur to drift upwards, backwards, and in outward rotation, either acutely or gradually.

624

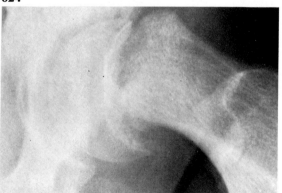

625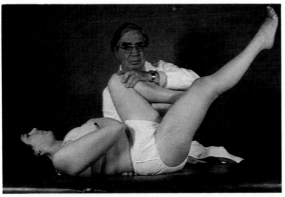

626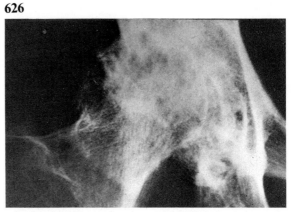

625 & 626   Osteoarthritis of the hip joint. This middle-aged lady had pain in the groin, buttock with referral to the right knee. She also had a limp. Thomas' test was positive, showing fixed flexion deformity of the right hip. The radiograph shows that she had severe degenerative osteoarthritis associated with segmental avascular necrosis of the femoral head. Its cause was undetermined.

627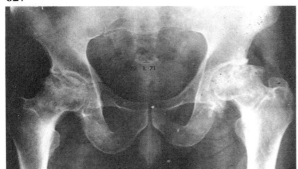

627   Avascular necrosis. Although the aetiology of osteoarthritis of the hip joint is uncertain in the majority of patients, a number of aetiological factors have been established. The radiograph showed typical bilateral osteoarthritis with patchy avascular necrosis in a severe alcoholic.

628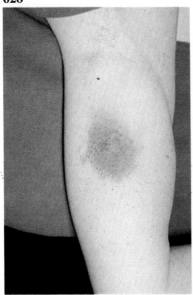

628 & 629   Thrombocytopenic purpura: a rare cause of osteoarthritis of the hip. There is marked loss of joint space and patchy avascular necrosis throughout the femoral heads, associated with impaired blood supply due to purpura.

629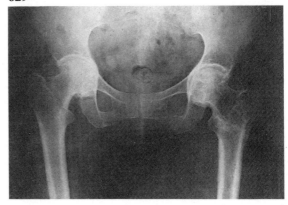

141

The knee joint

Rotational abnormalities of the lower limbs are chiefly due to the angle of anteversion of the femoral necks. In the foetus the femoral necks point almost directly forwards at 90°; by the time of birth the anteversion is 25°–30° and in adult life 16°–18°. Persistence of excessive anteversion of the femoral necks (PFA) is the usual cause of rotational deformity of the lower limbs.

630

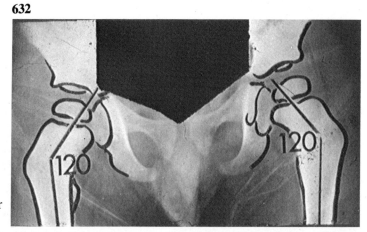

631

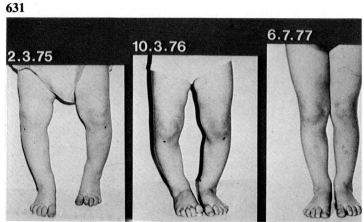

630 & 631   Genu varum. Physiological bow legs in a two year-old infant. Note the symmetry of the bowing. It is almost always due to transient abnormalities of rotation of the lower limbs. Bow legs under the age of three years are usually physiological and self-correcting.

632

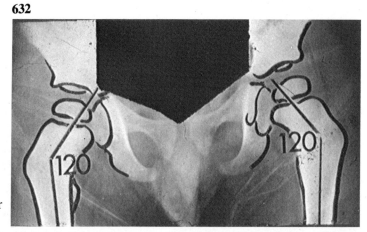

632   Normal neck-shaft angle of the upper end of the femora.

633

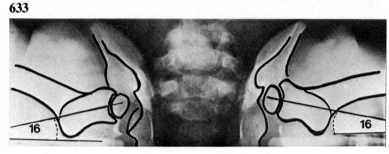

633   Normal anteversion angle of the femoral necks.

634

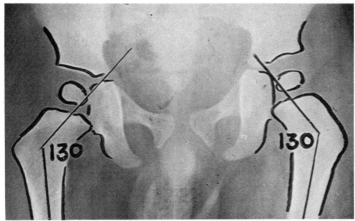

635

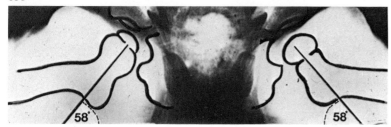

634 & 635 Although the anteroposterior view shows a neck-shaft angle within the normal range, the special projection lateral view, however, shows that the degree of anteversion of the femoral neck is in considerable excess of the normal.

636

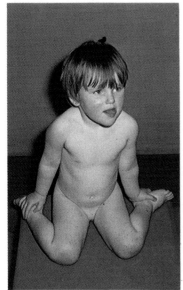

637

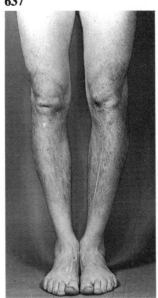

638

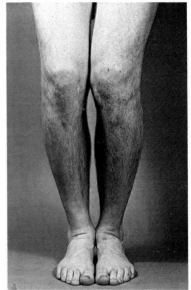

636 Persistent femoral anteversion. Children often elect to sit in this 'television position', comfortably locating their hips.

637 & 638 Apparent bow legs: this young man has apparent symmetrical bowing of his legs. When he slightly rotates his hips inwards, the apparent bowing disappears. It is due to persistent femoral anteversion.

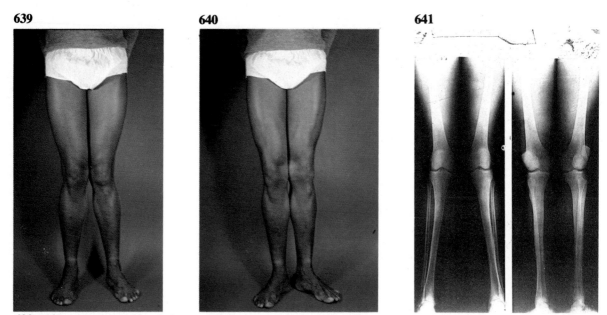

639–641 Apparent knock-knees: This young man's deformity disappears when he simply rotates his hips outwards. Note the position of the patellae. His knock-knees are due to an abnormality of anteversion of the femoral necks. In his case it is diminished.

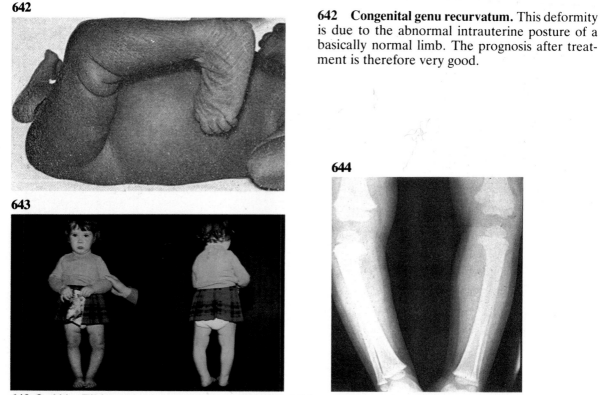

642 Congenital genu recurvatum. This deformity is due to the abnormal intrauterine posture of a basically normal limb. The prognosis after treatment is therefore very good.

643 & 644 Tibia vara. A very small number of children have bow legs which persist. They are usually children who have walked very early and the bowing is usually not symmetrical.
One leg is obviously more affected than the other. Distinctive 'beaking' on the medial side of the proximal tibial growth plates is apparent.

645

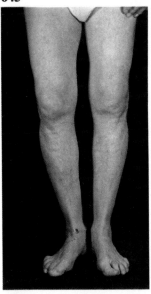

645 & 646   Genu varum in the adult. This man had straight legs and developed genu varum in middle age. The condition is unilateral. There is a history of a football injury 20 years previously causing degenerative arthritis affecting principally the medial compartment of the right knee – almost certainly secondary to an old meniscus injury.

646

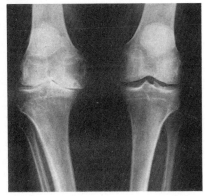

647

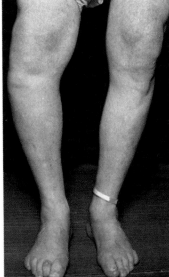

647 & 648   Post-traumatic genu varum following a major injury one year previously. The deformity is due to a malunited fracture of the upper end of the tibia and fibula.

648

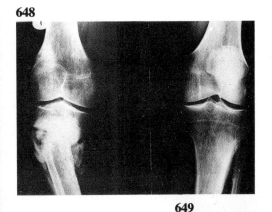

649

650

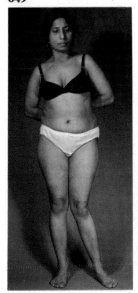

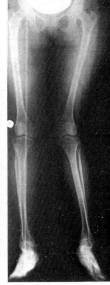

649 & 650   Unilateral genu valgum. No history of injury could be recalled, but the premature arrest on the lateral side of the upper tibial growth plate was almost certainly caused by a trivial injury.

651–654 **'Frame' knee.** This is now rarely seen as a complication of the treatment of tuberculosis of the hip on an abduction frame. There is general ligamentous laxity, and there may be premature epiphyseal arrest.

651 Anterior cruciate laxity indicated by 'anterior draw sign'.

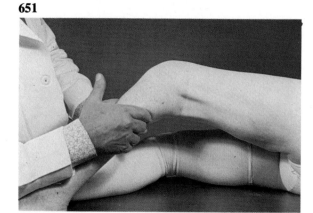

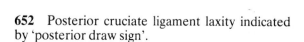

652 Posterior cruciate ligament laxity indicated by 'posterior draw sign'.

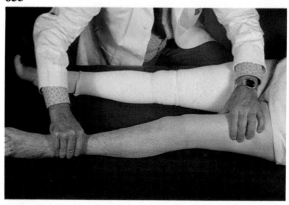

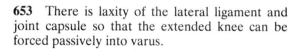

653 There is laxity of the lateral ligament and joint capsule so that the extended knee can be forced passively into varus.

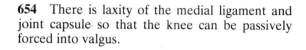

654 There is laxity of the medial ligament and joint capsule so that the knee can be passively forced into valgus.

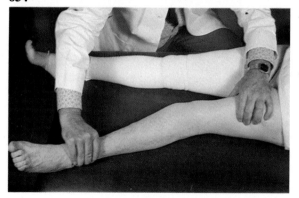

655

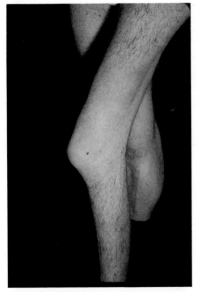

655 'Triple deformity' of the knee is seen as a consequence of muscle imbalance. It may follow poliomyelitis in childhood. The three deformities are posterior subluxation, external rotation and valgus.

656

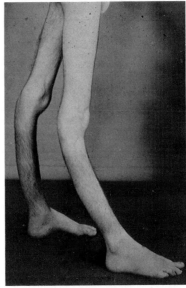

656 Genu recurvatum. This young man had an attack of poliomyelitis in infancy. In spite of the excessive extension of the knees, both quadriceps muscles are paralysed. He was able to stand with the knees locked back passively for stability. The deformity is of considerable advantage to the patient. It is either functionally acquired, or deliberately produced by surgery.

657

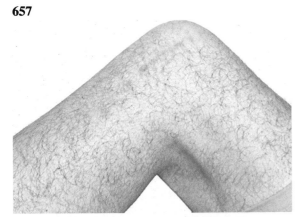

657–659 Chronic rupture of the anterior cruciate ligament of the knee. There is no abnormality seen with the knee in flexion at rest. The 'anterior drawer sign is markedly positive'.

658

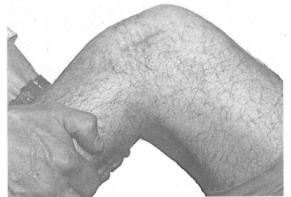

659

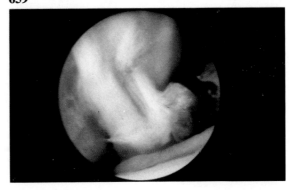

659 Disruption of the anterior cruciate ligament is seen on arthroscopy.

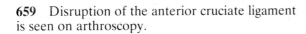

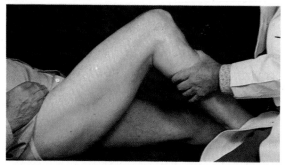

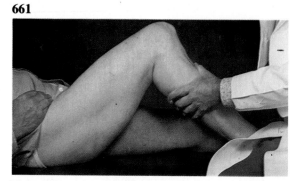

660 & 661 Chronic rupture of the posterior cruciate ligament. At rest in flexion the upper end of the tibia is subluxated backwards on the femur.

The subluxation is passively increased by backward pressure.

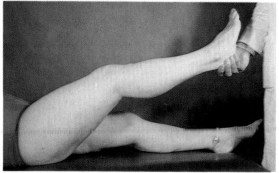

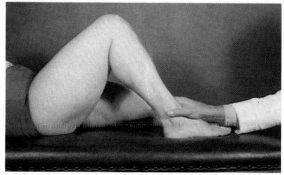

662 & 663 'Locked Knee'. This term is used to imply lack of normal extension of the knee following injury. With the leg hanging fully dependent on the examiner's hand, the knee stops some 20° short of full extension. It should be compared with the

opposite side. The knee is not truly locked because a good range of flexion remains. The locked knee may be due to a loose body, but it is usually due to injury to one or other meniscus.

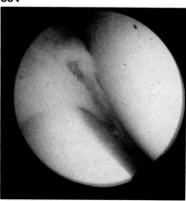

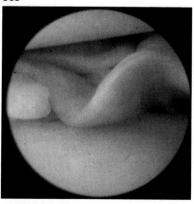

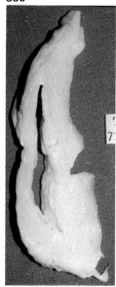

664–666 Ruptured medial meniscus. The arthrographic examination is seen in **664**, the arthroscopic examination in **665** and the operative specimen – 'bucket-handle' rupture in **666**.

667

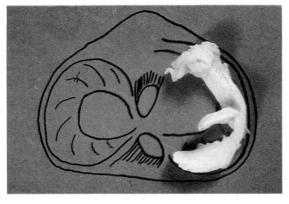

667 Ruptured medial meniscus, showing a posterior tag, one of the common varieties of medial meniscus rupture.

668

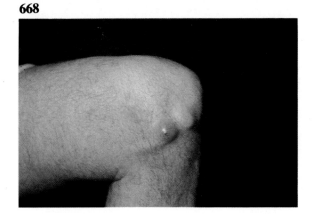

668 Multilocular cyst. Two soft swellings on the medial aspect of this man's left knee. They cause minimal pain and little impairment of function.

669

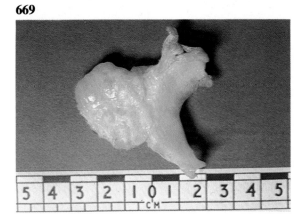

669 Multilocular cyst. Operative specimen to show arising from the perimeter of the medial meniscus.

670

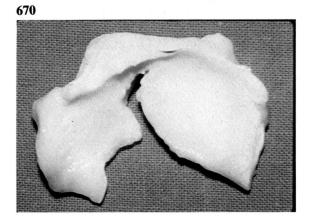

670 Rupture of lateral meniscus. This more often ruptures transversely. The pattern of such a transverse rupture can be structured like a parrot's beak.

671

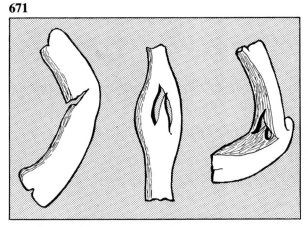

671 'Parrot-beak' rupture of the lateral meniscus.

672

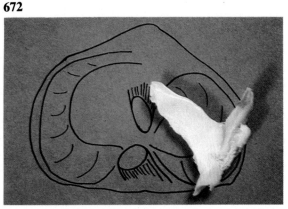

672 Another pattern of rupture of lateral meniscus causing locking of the knee.

673–676 Cyst of the lateral meniscus. This is at least six times more common than a cyst of the medial meniscus. There is often a history of previous injury.

673 A small lateral meniscus cyst can best be seen with the knee in the semiflexed position.

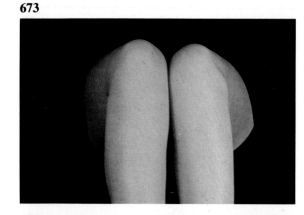

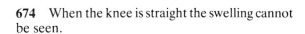

674 When the knee is straight the swelling cannot be seen.

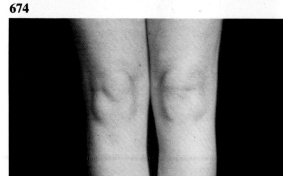

675 When the knee is fully flexed the swelling cannot be seen.

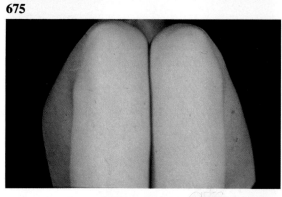

676 The lateral meniscus removed with its attached cyst.

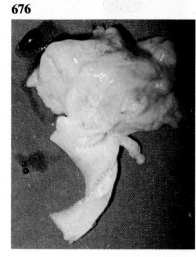

677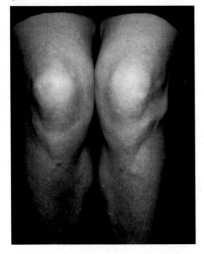

678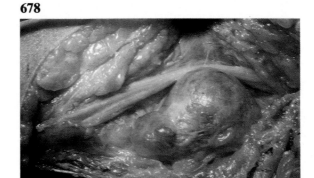

677–679 Multilocular ganglion. Swelling on the outer aspect of the left knee which does *not* disappear on full extension and flexion may be due to a ganglion arising from the superior tibiofibular joint. Multilocular ganglion is seen in close association with the common peroneal nerve.

679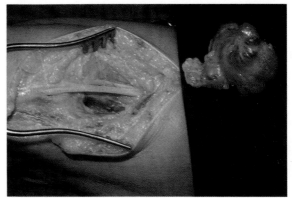

679 The ganglion is dissected free from the nerve.

680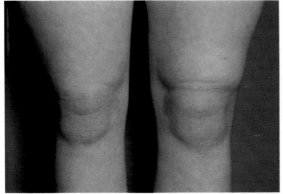

681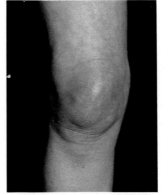

680 Rupture of the quadriceps muscle. This may occur after a trivial injury as the final insult in a degenerate tendon. It has been described as the presenting symptom in a patient suffering from diabetes or, classically, tabes dorsalis.

681 Prepatellar bursitis. Swelling of the prepatellar bursa may be due to occupational pressure, but 'housemaid's knee' affects the infrapatellar bursa which bears direct weight on kneeling.

682

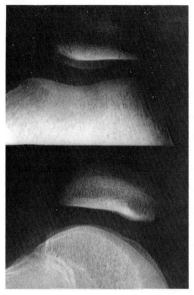

683

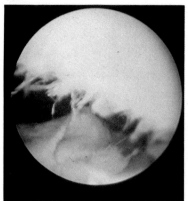

683 Fibrillation of articular cartilage seen through an arthroscope. Occasionally the condition becomes progressive and unequal pressures upon the articular cartilage of the patella produces pathological changes.

682–686 Chondromalacia patellae. Patellofemoral pain is a very common symptom, particularly in adolescent girls. It is probably due to transient mal-alignment of the extensor mechanism at the knee causing unequal pressure on the patellar facets.

684

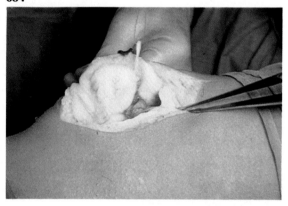

684 Condition of the patella seen at operation.

685

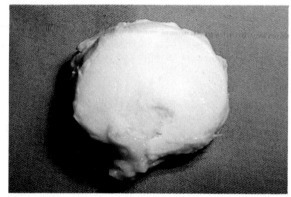

685 The lesion is initially almost entirely confined to one facet – usually the lateral.

686

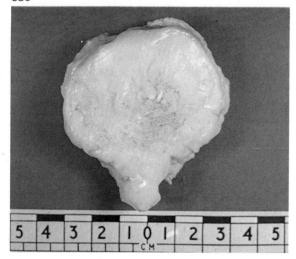

686 The entire articular surface of the patella has become involved in this more advanced case.

687

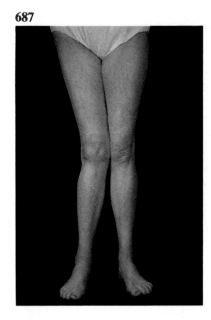

688

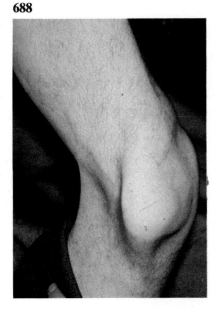

687 & 688 Patellar instability.
Post-traumatic unilateral genu valgum in a young girl leads to mal-alignment of the extensor mechanism and lateral instability of the patella. Recurrent dislocation of patella occurred.

689

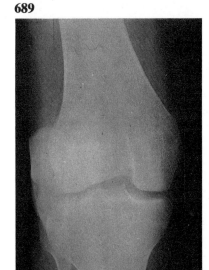

690

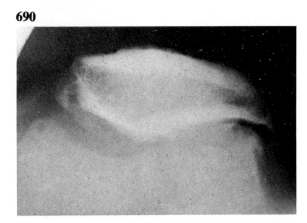

689 & 690 Radiograph taken at the time of dislocation. An anteroposterior radiograph shows the lateral dislocation. The skyline view shows degenerative changes in the patellofemoral joint, affecting principally, the lateral facet. Such changes are seen, either as the end result of chondromalacia patellae, or after recurrent dislocation of the patella.

691

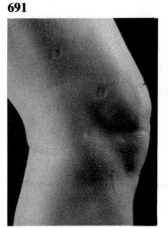

692

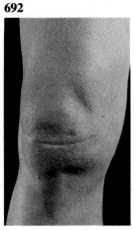

691 & 692 Excision of the patella. Note the virtually normal appearance of the knee apart from the scar. Patients are often unnecessarily concerned by the prospect of disfigurement from this operation.

693

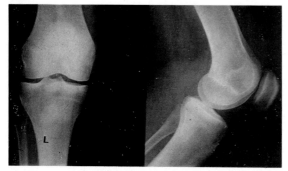

694

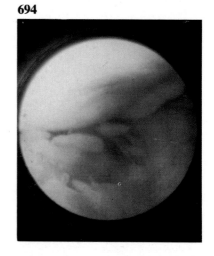

693–698 Synovial chondromatosis. The knees of a young man suffering from pain, swelling and repeated locking of the knee in which radiographs appear normal.

694 At arthroscopy multiple cartilagenous loose bodies can be seen.

695

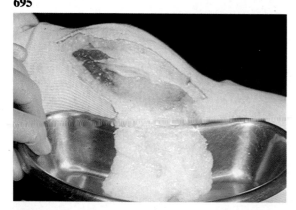

695 A large number of chondromata are removed at operation.

696

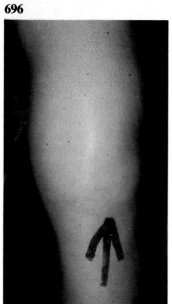

697

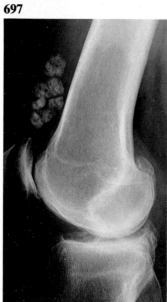

698

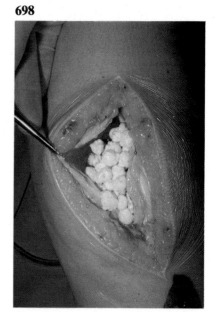

696–698 A gradual swelling of the knee developed in this patient. The radiograph revealed multiple chondromata. This is probably the same condition at a later stage when bone forms in several of the cartilage nodules.

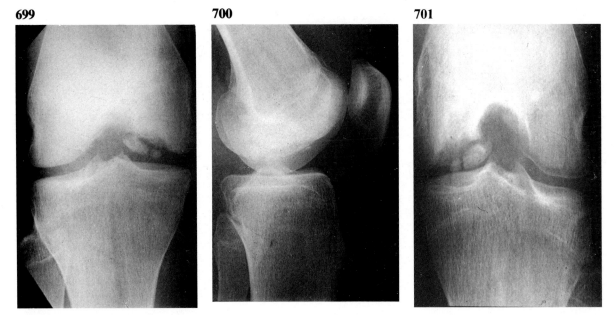

699–703   Osteochondritis dissecans. This condition may occur in several joints, but by far the commonest site is the lateral femoral condyle. Its aetiology is undefined. The lesion can be seen in the anteroposterior and lateral views but the extent of the lesion is best seen in the 'tunnel' view.

702

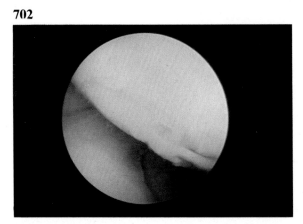

702   Osteochondritis dissecans seen through the arthroscope.

703   At operation the articular cartilage is seen to be separated with a minimal layer of subchondral bone and is eventually shed into the joint as a 'classical loose body'.

703

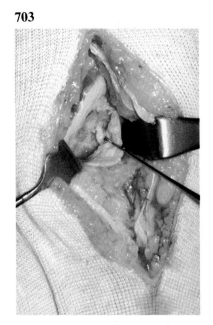

704

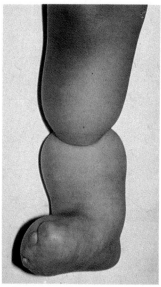

705

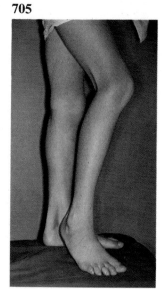

704 Congenital constriction ring. Rarely a limb is put at hazard by an amniotic band or the umbilical cord in utero. Here constriction has prejudiced the normal development of the limb distal to it.

705 Congenital contracture of the calf. Of the many causes of calf muscle shortening, possibly the least common is a simple congenital contracture of the calf muscle as is shown here. There are no associated abnormalities, and no cause is discernible.

706

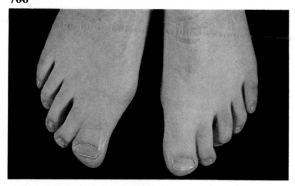

707

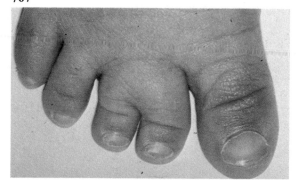

706 & 707 Syndactylism. Many varieties of syndactily occur varying from isolated fusion of two toes to widespread fusion of several digits of hand and foot.

708

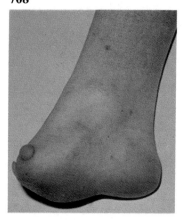

708 & 709 Congenital amputation of the forefoot. The fact that this is not due to a constriction ring is evidenced by the associated abnormalities of the hands. The aetiology is unknown.

709

710

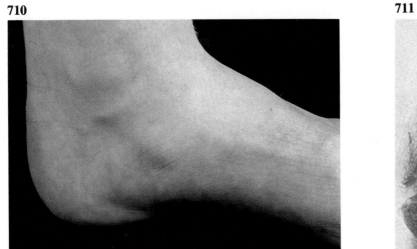

711

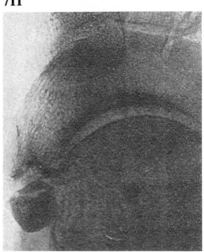

710 & 711   Os tibiale externum. This is one variety of several possible accessory tarsal ossicles. Although it is sited on the inner aspect of the foot, it derives its name from its position on the pre-axial border of the foetal limb bud.

712

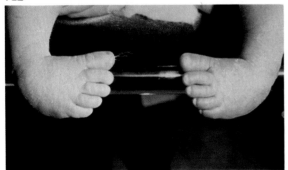

712   Congenital talipes equinovarus. The commonest variety of clubfoot, may be unilateral or bilateral; it may be postural or structural.

713

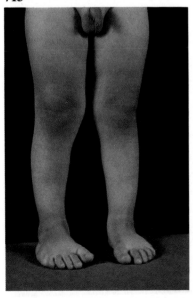

714

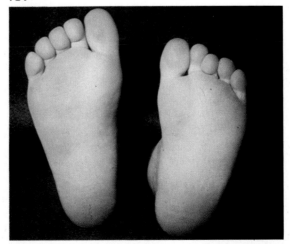

713 & 714   Talipes equino-varus: the residual deformity followed treatment which has not achieved full correction. The forefoot remains adducted. Note the shortening of the left foot and the inversion of the heel.

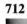

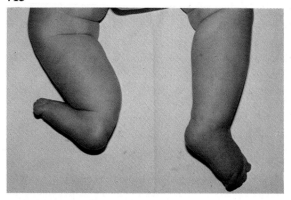

715 Congenital calcaneovalgus. This is the simplest variety of flatfoot. It is probably due to abnormal intrauterine posture. The foot is fundamentally normal and therefore responds readily to conservative treatment.

716 & 717 Congenital vertical talus. Extreme flatfoot position is due to a structural abnormality. Treatment is difficult and often unrewarding. The vertical position of the talus distinguishes this from simple calcaneovalgus flatfoot.

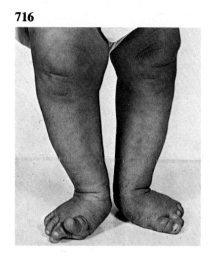

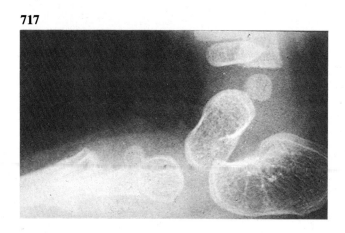

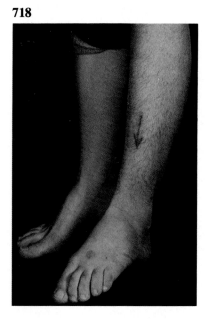

718 & 719 Spasmodic flatfoot. Also known as peroneal muscular spasm. A variety of flatfoot seen in the more mature person. It may be the presenting feature of any inflammatory disorder of the subtaloid joint; in a healthy individual it is due to a local structural abnormality. Radiograph shows a congenital bar of ossification between the calcaneus and navicular bones. Any variety of similar structural abnormality is the usual cause of spasmodic flatfoot in an otherwise healthy person.

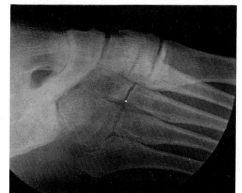

720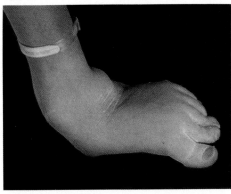

721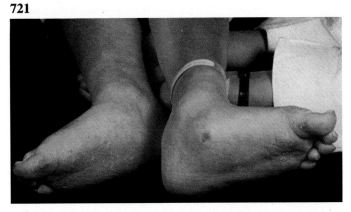

720 & 721   Pes planovalgus (flatfoot): an extreme example caused by rheumatoid arthritis leading to destructive arthropathy. Collapse of the medial arch of the foot. Whereas pressure ulceration is common in pes cavus, it is rare in pes planus.

722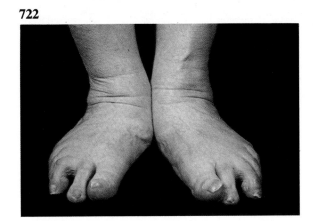

723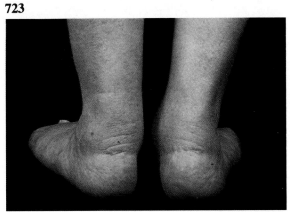

724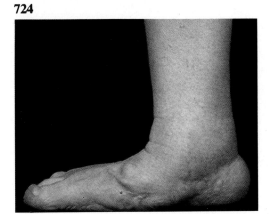

722–724   Postural flatfoot. The feet of an elderly and obese woman whose longitudinal arches have collapsed. These feet were fundamentally normal but have simply given way owing to increased body load and loss of muscle tone. From behind, the everted position of the heels can be seen. From the side the total collapse of the medial longitudinal arch is shown.

725

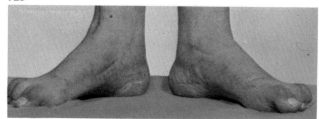

725 Pes cavus. The high arched foot has a deformity which is the opposite to flatfoot and is clinically the more significant and more important deformity. Contrary to common belief, it is the more serious of the two extremes. Pes cavus is often the local expression of some other disorder.

726

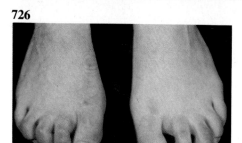

726 Clawing of the toes is usually associated with pes cavus.

727

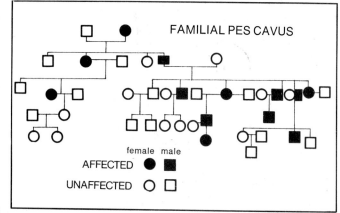

727 Familial pes cavus. There is a familial history in about 50% of patients with bilateral symmetrical pes cavus. The pattern shows that it is of autosomal dominant inheritance. It has been shown to be genetically linked to Friedreich's ataxia.

728

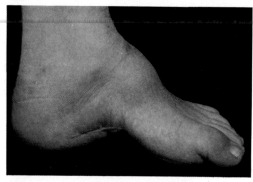

728 & 729 Friedreich's ataxia. The short stubby high-arched foot is characteristic in this disease. Both feet are affected more or less symmetrically.

729

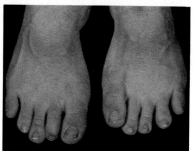

730

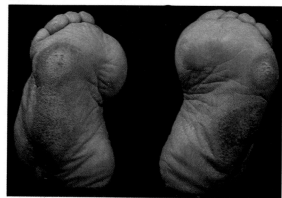

731

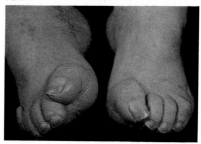

730 The feet of an older and more advanced case shows the very short foot, retracted toes, high medial arch and abnormal lateral weightbearing callosities.

731 Peroneal muscular dystrophy. (HMSN type I). Pes cavus and retraction of the toes is often the earliest sign of a slowly progressive hereditary motor neuron disease.

732

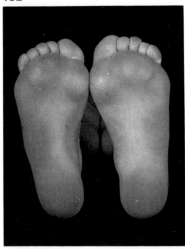

732 & 733 The feet of a young girl who complained of difficulty in obtaining comfortable shoes. Abnormal pressure points can be seen.

733

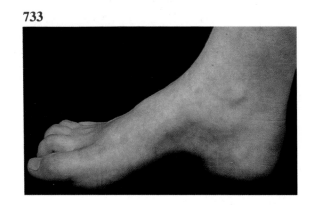

734

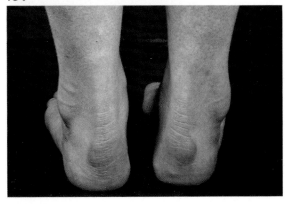

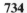

734 The back view of her feet show that the pes cavus is bilateral but not absolutely symmetrical, the right heel is more inverted.

735–737 Examination of her spine revealed a depression at the lumbosacral region with some abnormal discolouration of the skin. Anteroposterior radiograph showed spina bifida of L5 and a defect of the posterior wall of the sacrum; lateral radiograph showed that in addition to the posterior defect, a mild degree of spondylolisthesis was present. After further studies she was classified as a case of congenital spinal dysraphism.

735

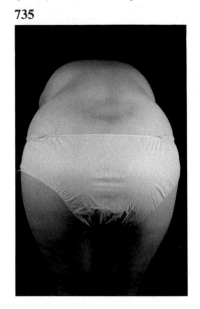

736

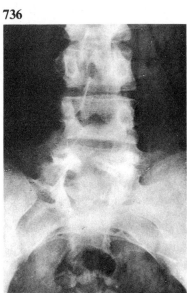

737

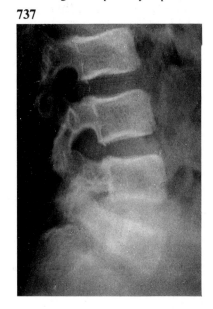

Poliomyelitis (see also 164–175)

738 Post-paralytic equinovarus, following an attack of poliomyelitis in childhood. The patient's left leg is shortened and his calf is contracted, causing him to stand in equinus. The heel is in varus.

739 Deformity due to muscle imbalance. The normally acting extensor hallucis longus in the presence of a paralysed tibialis anterior leads to imbalance in this patient's foot.

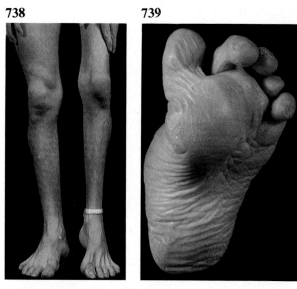

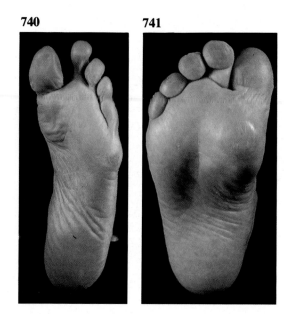

740 Pressure on the base of the 5th metatarsal bone is due to normally acting tibialis anterior and posterior muscles, when the peroneal muscles have been paralysed.

741 Excessive pressure on the head of the first metatarsal is due to a strongly acting peroneus longus when its antagonist, tibialis anterior, is paralysed.

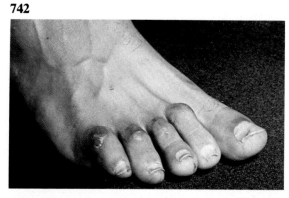

742 Clawing of the toes with secondary pressure on the PIP (proximal interphalangeal) joints is common. It is due to imbalance between normally acting extensor tendons of the toes when the intrinsic muscles are paralysed.

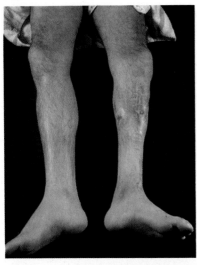

743

743 Volkmann's ischaemic contracture. This patient had a crush fracture of the left tibia and fibula. There is serious involvement of the posterior muscles which are wasted and contracted.

744 & 745 Ischaemic contracture of the long flexor muscles: when the ankle is passively dorsiflexed, the scarred long flexors force the toes into a fully flexed position; when the ankle is fully plantar flexed the toes can straighten.

745

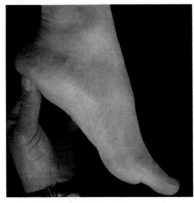

744

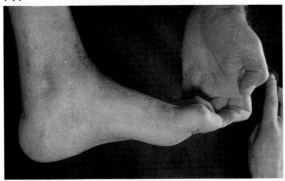

746

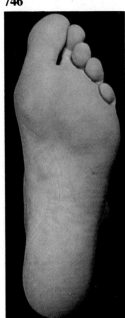

747

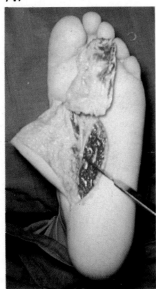

746 Fibrosis of the plantar fascia. Note the nodular thickening on the sole of the foot. The patient had Dupuytren's contracture of both hands. (See **511–513**)

747 The affected plantar fascia excised at operation.

748 Hammer toe. Only one or two toes on each foot are affected. There are a variety of deformities of the toe, depending at which joint the principal deformity is sited. The deformity is fixed. It is often familial.

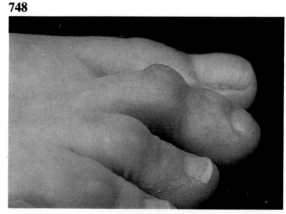

748

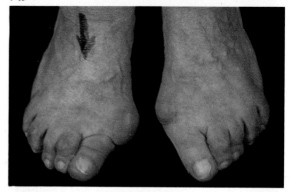

749 Hallux valgus. The angle subtended between the first metatarsal and the proximal phalanx is usually no more than about 10°. In this foot the angle is over 30°. The condition is often bilateral. An adventitious bursa over the prominent medial aspect of each metatarsal head has become enlarged and inflamed to form a bunion.

749

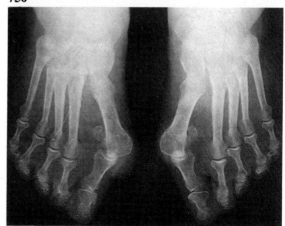

750 Metatarsus primus varus. The presumed cause of the hallux valgus shown in weight-bearing radiograph. It is due to a congenital abnormality of the first metatarsal bones which are in excessive varus: metatarsus primus varus. It is a condition of sex-linked autosomal inheritance.

750

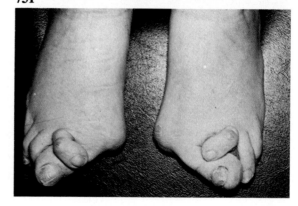

751 Hallux valgus: a more advanced case with bunions and overriding of the adjacent second toes. Note not only the severe valgus deformity, but also the considerable rotation of the big toes, the nails of which now look medially.

751

164

752

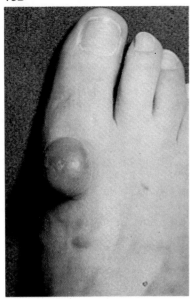

753

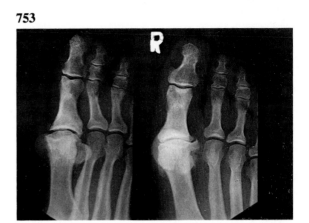

752 & 753 Hallux rigidus. The inflamed bunion in hallux rigidus occurs not on the medial but on the dorsal aspect of the head of the first metatarsal bone.

753 Radiographs show arthritic changes of the first metatarsophalangeal joint and the dorsal exostosis.

754

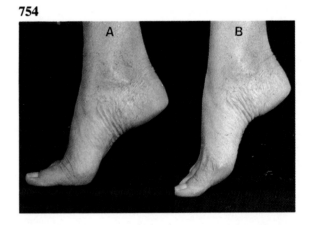

754 Hallux rigidus. In normal walking, the 'take-off' occurs at the metatarsophalangeal joint of the big toe which must therefore dorsiflex (**A**). If it cannot do so the 'take-off' now occurs at the inter-phalangeal joint which is forced to hyperextend beyond the stiff MP metatarsophalangeal joint (**B**).

755

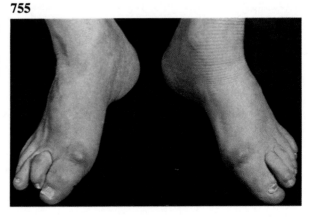

755 Bunion due to gout. This is the classical but by no means the commonest presentation of gout. Note the absence of any hallux valgus. The bunion is due to the deposition of uric acid crystals in the bursa.

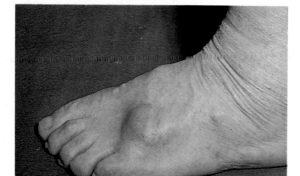

3 Miscellaneous

756 Recurrent ganglion of the ankle. This swelling was thought to be a ganglion arising from the tibialis anterior tendon sheath. At the second excision it was noted to arise from the ankle joint.

757 Soft-tissue tumour on the dorsum of the foot which turned out to be a xanthoma of the synovial tendon sheath of the toes.

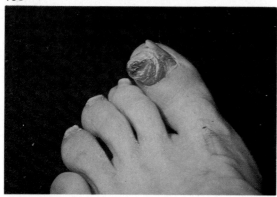

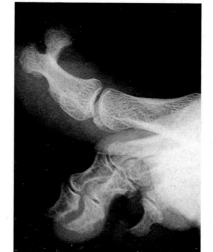

758 & 759 Subungual exostosis may develop on the dorsum of the terminal phalanx, usually of the great toe, and present as a derangement of nail growth. It is probably due to preceding trauma.

760

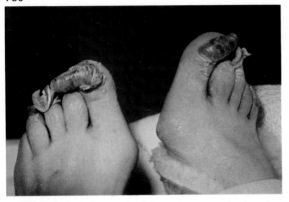

760 Onychogryposis. An unsightly but harmless condition due to deformed overgrowth of the nails. Also known as 'Ram's horn nail'.

761

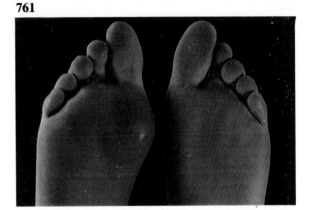

761 Simple calcified bursa. This patient presented with a painful swelling under the head of the right first metatarsal.

762

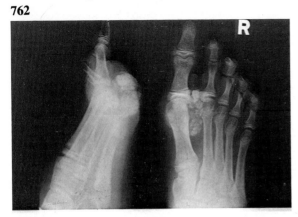

762 Calcification independent of the sesamoid bones.

763

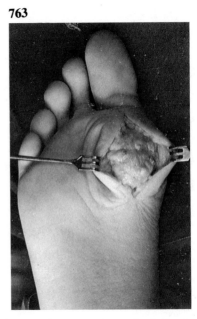

763 At operation a solid mass unattached to any important structure was removed and on section showed to be a simple calcified bursa.

764

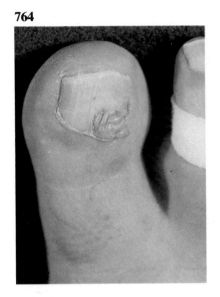

764 Simple verucca. It is important to distinguish this from a malignant melanoma which may be non-pigmented.

765

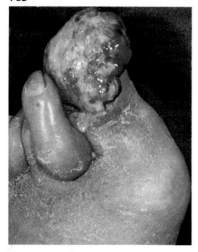

765   Malignant epithelioma.

766

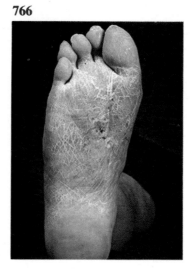

767

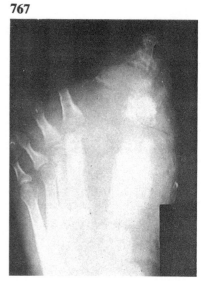

766 & 767   Madura foot. The patient had an indurated wound with intermittent discharge for seven years on the sole of his left foot. Investigation established the diagnosis as due to infection by the mycetoma fungus.

768

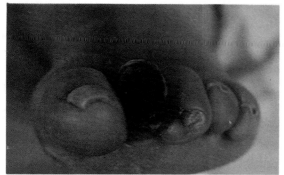

768   Gangrene of the second toe due to peripheral vascular disease.

769

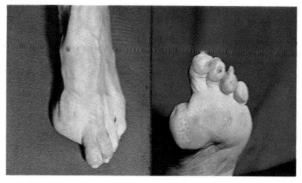

769   Frostbite. Gangrene forced an amputation of the big toe. The other toes are wasted and retracted due to paralysis of the intrinsic musculature.

770

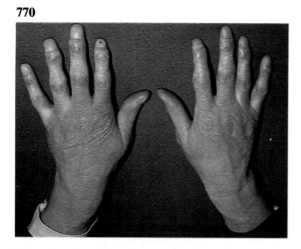

770   The hands of the same patient also affected by cold.

771

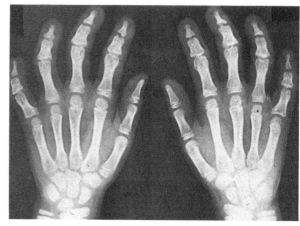

771   Changes which developed in the phalanges after frostbite.

Index

Numbers refer to pages